Coping with Asthma in Adults

Mark Greener spent a decade in biomedical research before joining *MIMS Magazine* for GPs in 1989. Since then, he's written on health and biology or magazines worldwide for non-specialists, healthcare professionals and scientists. He's the author of nine other books and lives with his wife, three children and two cats in a Cambridgeshire village.

Overcoming Common Problems Series

Selected titles

A full list of titles is available from Sheldon Press,
36 Causton Street, London SW1P 4ST and on our website at
www.sheldonpress.co.uk

101 Questions to Ask Your Doctor
Dr Tom Smith

Asperger Syndrome in Adults
Dr Ruth Searle

The Assertiveness Handbook
Mary Hartley

Assertiveness: Step by step
Dr Windy Dryden and Daniel Constantinou

Backache: What you need to know
Dr David Delvin

Body Language: What you need to know
David Cohen

Bulimia, Binge-eating and their Treatment
Professor J. Hubert Lacey, Dr Bryony Bamford
and Amy Brown

The Cancer Survivor's Handbook
Dr Terry Priestman

The Chronic Pain Diet Book
Neville Shone

Cider Vinegar
Margaret Hills

Coeliac Disease: What you need to know
Alex Gazzola

Confidence Works
Gladeana McMahon

Coping Successfully with Pain
Neville Shone

Coping Successfully with Prostate Cancer
Dr Tom Smith

Coping Successfully with Psoriasis
Christine Craggs-Hinton

Coping Successfully with Ulcerative Colitis
Peter Cartwright

Coping Successfully with Varicose Veins
Christine Craggs-Hinton

Coping Successfully with Your Hiatus Hernia
Dr Tom Smith

Coping Successfully with Your Irritable Bowel
Rosemary Nicol

Coping When Your Child Has Cerebral Palsy
Jill Eckersley

Coping with Age-related Memory Loss
Dr Tom Smith

**Coping with Birth Trauma and Postnatal
Depression**
Lucy Jolin

Coping with Bowel Cancer
Dr Tom Smith

Coping with Bronchitis and Emphysema
Dr Tom Smith

Coping with Candida
Shirley Trickett

Coping with Chemotherapy
Dr Terry Priestman

Coping with Chronic Fatigue
Trudie Chalder

Coping with Coeliac Disease
Karen Brody

Coping with Compulsive Eating
Dr Ruth Searle

**Coping with Diabetes in Childhood
and Adolescence**
Dr Philippa Kaye

Coping with Diverticulitis
Peter Cartwright

Coping with Dyspraxia
Jill Eckersley

Coping with Early-onset Dementia
Jill Eckersley

**Coping with Eating Disorders
and Body Image**
Christine Craggs-Hinton

Coping with Envy
Dr Windy Dryden

**Coping with Epilepsy in Children
and Young People**
Susan Elliot-Wright

Coping with Family Stress
Dr Peter Cheevers

Coping with Gout
Christine Craggs-Hinton

Coping with Hay Fever
Christine Craggs-Hinton

Coping with Headaches and Migraine
Alison Frith

Coping with Hearing Loss
Christine Craggs-Hinton

Overcoming Common Problems

Coping with Asthma in Adults

MARK GREENER

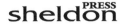

First published in Great Britain in 2011

Sheldon Press
36 Causton Street
London SW1P 4ST
www.sheldonpress.co.uk

British Library Cataloguing-in-Publication Data

A catalogue record for this book is available from the British Library

ISBN 978–1–84709–156–7

Typeset by Kenneth Burnley Studios, Wirral, Cheshire
First printed in Great Britain by Ashford Colour Press
Subsequently digitally printed in Great Britain

Produced on paper from sustainable forests

Contents

As always:
to Rose, Yasmin, Rory and Ophelia.

Introduction

For many people, asthma evokes images of wheezing, breathless children puffing away on inhalers in playgrounds. However, according to the charity Asthma UK, around four in every five asthma sufferers are adults. Doctors in the UK currently treat around 1.1 million children for asthma – and 4.3 million adults.

Some of these adults have had asthma since childhood. Some were asthmatic as kids, but their symptoms faded during adolescence, only to resurface in later life. Others developed asthma for the first time as adults – even into their 70s and 80s. Indeed, around 700,000 people over the age of 65 years live with asthma across the UK. As we'll see, coping with asthma when you're elderly can prove particularly difficult.

Furthermore, the number of adults with asthma is rising. Doctors now regard some adults previously diagnosed with chronic obstructive pulmonary disease (COPD) and children once regarded as suffering from 'wheezy bronchitis' as asthmatic. Even allowing for such changing diagnostic fashions, the number of asthma cases increased markedly over the last few decades of the twentieth century. So, the numbers of adults with asthma will increase over the next few years as asthmatic children reach middle age and beyond. Meanwhile, the increasing number of elderly people in the population will probably drive a rise in the number of cases of late-onset asthma.

Apart from being more common, asthma in adults is often more serious than in children. Adults are much more likely than their younger counterparts to die from asthma. Every premature death is a tragedy. Fortunately, effective modern drugs mean that deaths from asthma are rare, especially in view of the millions of people who suffer from the disease in the UK. Nevertheless, one person dies from asthma in the UK every seven hours – and most are adults. During 2008, 29 of the 1,204 people who died from asthma in the UK were aged 14 years or under. More than two-thirds of deaths from asthma occurred in people over 65 years of age. Adults also account for 58 per cent of hospital admissions for asthma. Tragically, Asthma UK comment, better care could prevent up to 90 per cent of deaths and 75 per cent of hospital admissions due to asthma.

Problems at home, at work and at play

More commonly, poorly managed asthma undermines almost every aspect of adult life. According to Asthma UK, 61 per cent of people with asthma say that their asthma stops them from getting a good night's sleep, while 42 per cent of people with allergies (one cause of asthma) say that the disease undermines their social life. Furthermore, up to 90 per cent of people with asthma suffer symptoms when they exercise, which can stop people jogging, taking part in sport or working out in the gym. So, asthma indirectly increases the risk of, for example, obesity (a risk factor for severe asthma) and heart disease. Exercise-induced asthma can even hinder a satisfying sex life. Much of this suffering is unnecessary: effective treatment can prevent exercise-induced symptoms. Indeed, many elite athletes would, if untreated, experience exercise-induced symptoms.

As a final example of asthma's malevolent influence on adults' lives: work-related factors probably cause up to a quarter of asthma cases among adults and contribute to approximately 15 per cent of severe attacks (the medical term is 'exacerbations'). My own asthma symptoms really took hold – and my doctor diagnosed the disease – when I was in my 20s. A combination of factors at work and the mould in our Victorian terraced house probably triggered my attacks, several of which ended in frightening trips to accident and emergency (A&E) departments. However, in retrospect, I had experienced symptoms before: As a child I often had a nagging cough, which I put down to my father's addiction to foul-smelling pipes and small cigars, and I became more breathless than I should have during school sports.

Unfortunately, work-related asthma often prompts unwanted career changes. More commonly, asthma causes sick leave, which may hinder prospects in an increasingly competitive job market. A survey by Asthma UK found that 21 per cent of asthmatics had taken between one and five days off sick because of asthma during the year before the study. Five per cent took more than six days' sick leave.

However, coping with asthma using drugs and the other approaches outlined in this book can improve your work life. An American study, published in the *Journal of Asthma*, reported that 43 per cent of adults with uncontrolled asthma had missed work in the previous six months, compared to 24 per cent of those with well-controlled symptoms. (You can find details of the studies mentioned in the book in References, pp. 124–30.) Adults with uncontrolled asthma missed twice as many days from work as their better-managed counterparts: on average, six and three days in the previous six months, respectively.

Nevertheless, asthma still accounts for 12.7 million lost days at work and costs the UK economy £1.2 billion each year. Asthma caused by work-related factors alone costs the UK economy between £95 million and £135 million annually. Nevertheless, patients, rather than employers or the government, shoulder almost half the economic burden imposed by occupational asthma through, for example, lost earnings.

Adult asthma: a neglected disease?

Despite being common, potentially deadly and expensive, asthma in adults rarely receives the attention it deserves. For example, asthma's underlying mechanism may change as we age: in particular, allergies are a much more common cause of asthma in children than in adults. Although the 'classic' cause of asthma, allergies appear to account for, at most, only half of asthma cases in adults. Nevertheless, relatively few studies examine asthma caused by factors other than allergy. And despite their increased risk of severe asthma and serious exacerbations, relatively few studies examine the cells and molecules that drive asthma in adults generally and in the elderly in particular. Understanding these basic biological drivers is essential in the search for new treatments.

Furthermore, much of the information about asthma management comes from studies that included children with allergic asthma. Indeed, many studies of asthma treatments specifically exclude patients older than 65 years of age or those with other diseases (so-called co-morbidities), which simplifies analysis of the results and may protect volunteers from side effects. After all, at least half of people 65 years and over have three or more co-morbidities, several of which (such as some heart conditions and COPD) can complicate the diagnosis and management of asthma. However, such exclusions make it difficult for doctors to extrapolate from the young person with asthma alone in the study to the older patient in their clinic with several diseases.

The lack of specific evidence helps explain why, despite a growing range of treatments, asthma in adults often remains poorly managed. In a large study called INSPIRE, adults with asthma experienced, on average, an exacerbation every month (11.8 a year) and 27 per cent of these exacerbations were severe. Even people reporting well-controlled asthma experienced, on average, just over six exacerbations annually. This study underscores that asthma patients often have low expectations of treatment. Suffering an exacerbation every two months means that the asthma is, arguably, not well controlled.

Finally, despite asthma markedly impairing adults' lives, despite the distressing symptoms, despite the risk of death and disability, many older people don't see their GP when they experience asthmatic symptoms. Many adults seem to regard breathlessness as part of the inevitable price we pay for growing old and in many cases limit their activities rather than changing treatment.

This book focuses on the particular problems and issues facing adults as they try to cope with asthma. We'll consider the diagnosis and the triggers for asthma in adults, many of which (occupational factors, pregnancy and the menopause, to take three obvious examples) differ from those in children. We'll explore the drugs and other approaches adults can take to control their symptoms, enrich their quality of life and perform the activities of daily life that everyone else seems to take for granted to live full, active and satisfying lives.

Note: This book is not intended to replace advice from your doctor. You should always consult your doctor if you are experiencing symptoms with which you feel you need help.

1

What is asthma?

Asthma is one of the most common diseases among adults. According to Asthma UK, doctors currently treat around 4.3 million adults for asthma. Of these, 700,000 are over the age of 65 years. Those figures are sobering enough. However, many cases of asthma among adults, especially in older people, remain undiagnosed.

Two main factors are largely responsible for the under-diagnosis. First, asthma's symptoms overlap with several other conditions, which complicates diagnosis (as we will see in Chapter 5). Second, older people who feel breathless or wheezy may not seek their doctor's help, mistakenly regarding the symptoms as the inevitable price of growing older. However, breathlessness and wheeze are certainly not always age-related: they're often signs of asthma, COPD or another disease (see Chapter 5). So, it's important to get yourself checked if you start wheezing or feeling breathless.

Asthma's natural history

Against this background, asthma's natural history in adults tends to follow one of three routes. Estimates vary from study to study, but between 30 and 80 per cent of adults with asthma have suffered from the disease since childhood. Others develop asthma for the first time as adults. In one study, by Loerbroks and colleagues, almost one in 50 (1.8 per cent) of a group of people aged between 40 and 65 years developed asthma over, on average, 8.5 years.

The final group experienced wheeze and other asthma symptoms when they were children, then recovered during adolescence only for the condition to re-emerge in later life. Recurrence of childhood symptoms is probably as common as new cases of asthma among adults. Of course, some people may not recall that they suffered asthma as a child. In other cases of 'adult-onset asthma', myself included, hindsight reveals possible symptoms during childhood. So, gaining an accurate picture is difficult. Nevertheless, to understand why some adults suffer from asthma and how we can cope with the disease, we need to start by looking at a healthy pair of lungs.

Inside our lungs

Unless something goes wrong – or we pant after running for a bus or after the kids in the park – we rarely think much about breathing. Respiration is one bodily function – like the beating of our heart – that remains remarkably reliable throughout life, even without conscious control. However, we consciously control breathing when we speak, sing or hold our breath.

At rest, we typically breathe 12 to 20 times each minute. The normal tidal volume – the amount of air that moves in and out of our lungs during inspiration and expiration when we do not make any extra effort – is around 500 ml. A normal pair of adult lungs can expel between 3 and 5 litres of air (vital capacity) after taking the deepest breath we can.

Our lungs do not expand fully each time we take a breath: we only use a small fraction of our vital capacity during each breath. A quarter of the air we inhale remains in the airways that connect the mouth and the alveoli (see below), where we exchange toxic carbon dioxide for the oxygen our cells need to remain alive, repair damage and divide.

Almost all cells contain mitochondria – essentially the cell's power-house. Mitochondria use oxygen to generate a chemical called adenosine triphosphate (ATP), the fuel for the cell's various activities. Without a steady supply of ATP, the processes that keep cells alive grind to a halt, and eventually the cell dies.

As everyone knows, you have two lungs: one on the left of your body, the other on the right. The left lung lies over your heart. So, the right lung is slightly larger and has three sections (lobes), while the smaller left lung consists of two lobes. Your ribcage surrounds and protects the spongy, fragile lungs and anchors some of the muscles you use to breathe (see Figure 1.1).

Muscles and breathing

Usually, you rely on two sets of muscles to breathe: the diaphragm and the intercostals:

- The diaphragm – a thick sheet of muscle – lies under the lungs, anchored to the lower part of the ribcage, the base of the sternum (breastbone) and the spine.
- The intercostal muscles run between each rib.

Underneath the ribs, two thin moist membranes – the pleura – cover each lung. These membranes slide over each other when you exhale and inhale. ('Pleurisy' refers to an inflammation of the pleura usually following an infection, such as flu.)

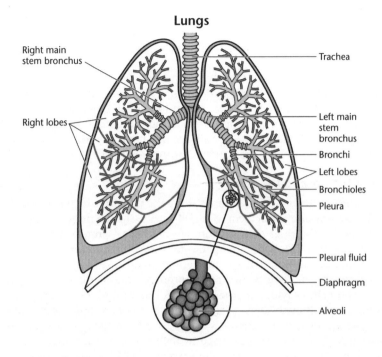

Lungs

Right main stem bronchus

Trachea

Right lobes

Left main stem bronchus

Bronchi

Left lobes

Bronchioles

Pleura

Pleural fluid

Diaphragm

Alveoli

Figure 1.1 Anatomy of the lungs

When relaxed, the diaphragm is dome-shaped. When you inhale, your diaphragm contracts and flattens. Meanwhile, the intercostals contract and shorten. Together, the two sets of muscles pull the ribcage up and out, which increases the space in the chest. So, the pressure inside the airways is lower than that outside. As a result, air flows through your mouth and nose, along your windpipe (trachea) and into your lungs. The diaphragm and intercostals then relax. The lungs and chest wall are elastic, so when the muscles relax the chest springs back to its original shape. This expels the air in the lungs, now rich in carbon dioxide.

Several other muscles aid breathing, especially when you exercise. For example:

- Three pairs of neck muscles, called the scalenes, lift and help expand the ribcage during inspiration (breathing in).
- The sternocleidomastoids, which connect your head to your shoulder, aid breathing especially during exercise and stress.
- Even if you don't have a six-pack, your abdominal muscles are very powerful. (They have to be strong to resist the pressure exerted by

the intestines and stop your belly from bulging outwards.) During rigorous exercise, abdominal muscles contract, which pushes the diaphragm against the lungs and expels more air.

Many people do not use their breathing muscles correctly – as you'll soon find out if you learn meditation, tai chi or one of the other martial arts. Most people have sufficient lung reserve to overcome their bad habits. However, in people with asthma this 'improper use' can exacerbate their symptoms. As we'll see in Chapter 7, you may be able to retrain your muscles and correct dysfunctional breathing.

From the nose to the alveoli

After the mouth and nose, air flows along the trachea, which is about 10 to 16 cm long and about 2 cm wide. Horseshoe-shaped rings of cartilage – rather like the rings on a vacuum cleaner hose – protect the trachea from crushing. The body's temperature warms the air as it travels. (As we'll see, cold air is one of the most common asthma triggers.)

The trachea forks into two major bronchi, one to each lung. Each major bronchus divides another 10 to 25 times into bronchi and then bronchioles. Bronchi have cartilage to strengthen their walls and support the airways. The final few branches of the respiratory tree, called bronchioles, do not have cartilage in their walls, and together end in between 300 million and 500 million alveoli. Each alveolus, which looks like a cauliflower floret, is about 0.1 to 0.2 mm in diameter (Figure 1.2). As they lack cartilage, bronchioles and alveoli rely on the surrounding tissues for the support they need to remain open. (Emphysema – a debilitating form of COPD – destroys these delicate tissues, as we'll see in Chapter 5.)

The bronchial tree's shape packs a vast area into a relatively small volume. Overall, our lungs contain approximately 1,500 miles of airways. In an adult, the alveoli's surface area is about 70 m² – roughly the same as a single tennis court. A network of around 620 miles of capillaries – small, thin blood vessels – surrounds the alveoli (Fig. 1.2). Oxygen dissolves in the fluid covering the thin alveoli and crosses into the bloodstream. Red blood cells (erythrocytes) pick up and carry oxygen to the tissues around your body.

Red blood cells collect some of the 'waste' carbon dioxide produced by cells, which they transport back to the lungs. However, 90 per cent of the carbon dioxide produced during respiration reaches the lungs dissolved, or combined with water, in blood.

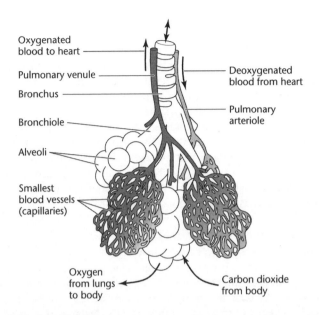

Figure 1.2 The alveoli

Anaemia and breathlessness

People with anaemia have too little haemoglobin, the iron-containing protein in red blood cells that carries oxygen. Some anaemic people produce too few red blood cells. Each red blood cell survives for 100 to 120 days, and the body destroys old, inefficient erythrocytes. However, in some anaemic patients the body destroys too many red blood cells, including some that are healthy and efficient. Numerous factors can trigger anaemia, such as deficiencies in vitamin B_{12} or iron, chronic inflammation and certain malignancies.

Anaemia's symptoms arise from a mismatch between the demand for oxygen by tissues and the supply by haemoglobin. As a result, an anaemic person may feel fatigued and weak or suffer headaches, chest pains and palpitations. If an anaemic person breathes normally, his or her body 'senses' that oxygen levels are too low. So, he or she feels breathless – a trigger to inhale more oxygen – and exercise becomes more difficult. Anaemia is one of several conditions that doctors may need to rule out when determining whether someone has asthma.

Our bodies need to keep levels of oxygen and carbon dioxide within tight limits. The respiratory centre at the base of the brain controls our breathing subconsciously. Sensors in the brain and certain blood vessels (aorta and carotid arteries) detect changes in levels of carbon dioxide and oxygen in the blood. Increased levels of carbon dioxide trigger us to breathe more rapidly and deeply. When carbon dioxide levels decline, we breathe less frequently and more shallowly.

However, the breathing of older people – even if they don't suffer from asthma or another lung disease – tends to show a less marked response to decreased oxygen and increased carbon dioxide levels than is typical among younger people. This impaired response is one of several age-related changes in our breathing that form the backdrop against which adult asthma develops.

Age-related changes in breathing

As you get older, almost every organ in your body changes – and your lungs are no exception. For example, age-related changes to the larynx (voice box) probably altered your voice's pitch, loudness and quality over the years. As you age, your voice may become quieter, slightly hoarse and 'weaker'. With age the pitch usually deepens in women and rises in men.

The lung matures until about a woman reaches about 20 and a man around 25 years of age. During childhood, lungs grow by increasing the number of bronchioles and alveoli. However, most of our complement of alveoli has emerged by around ten years of age and relatively few develop during adolescence. After our mid-20s, alveoli numbers decline. Obviously, this reduces the surface area available for gas exchange. While the decline in alveoli number is inevitable, environmental factors – especially smoking – can speed their destruction.

Muscles also weaken with age. As this includes your diaphragm and intercostals, older people typically generate less force during inspiration. Our chest and lungs also become less elastic, partly because we produce less 'elastin'. As this protein's name suggests, elastin allows skin, tendons, ligaments and other tissues to spring back into their 'normal' shape after stretching or contracting. In the lungs, the elastic recoil helps force air from the airways when we exhale. So, we drive air from the lungs less forcibly as we age.

Meanwhile, changes in bones and muscles often increase the depth of the chest. For example, along with the rest of the skeleton, bone mass in the ribs and vertebrae declines as we age, which predisposes to osteoporosis (brittle bone disease) and so increases the risk of breaking a bone. Oral steroids – used to treat asthma – can hasten the decline in our skeletal strength (Chapter 6). These and other age-related changes can alter the shape of the spine and the chest is less able to stretch during breathing.

Measurements of lung function (Chapter 5) reflect these age-related changes. For example, the rate at which air flows through the bronchi declines after around 30 years of age, and vital capacity (the maximum amount of air you can exhale) peaks around the age of 20 years and then falls by around 250 cc each decade. Fortunately, we normally have more lung function than we need for most activities. This 'reserve' means that elderly people should still be able to perform the activities of daily life. Indeed, many people still breathe reasonably well after having one of their lungs surgically removed.

Nevertheless, these age-related changes help to explain why asthma and other lung diseases can pose a particular problem for adults. One study compared two groups of otherwise similar asthma patients. One group was aged, on average, 35 years. The other group – whose average age was 60 years – showed a greater variation in peak flow (a measure of lung function, see Chapter 5) over the course of the day. This suggests that their asthma control was worse than that of their younger counterparts. The older people also reported more symptoms during the night – another indicator of poor control.

The age-related changes also help explain why childhood asthma can re-emerge in middle-aged or elderly adults despite disappearing during adolescence. Young children may not have enough lung reserve to cope with mild airway obstruction, so they suffer asthmatic symptoms. As they reach adolescence and young adulthood, improved lung function compensates for mild airway obstruction and the symptoms seem to resolve. But lung function declines as they age and symptoms re-emerge in later life.

Symptoms of asthma

The term 'asthma' derives from an ancient Greek word meaning 'breathless' or 'breathing with an open mouth'. Ancient Greeks used the term more widely than to describe only the constellation of symptoms (recurrent bouts of coughing, wheezing, chest tightness and breathlessness) we now call asthma.

While doctors first described the symptoms of asthma millennia ago, the cause remained largely a mystery until the twentieth century. We now know that allergies and several other factors trigger excessive inflammation in the lungs. This inflammation contracts the ring of muscles around the airways, which narrows the bronchi and bronchioles (Fig. 1.3). The narrowing obstructs the flow of air as we breathe in and out. Airway inflammation occurs at all stages of asthma, from newly diagnosed people with mild symptoms to those dying from intractable asthma. Indeed, the lungs remain inflamed even when the person is symptom-free. But as the inflammation increases in intensity, the severity of the symptoms worsens. (See Figure 1.3.)

The airway obstruction in asthma is largely reversible, as the attack abates or with treatment. But as you get older, the chance that the airway obstruction will not be totally reversible increases (we'll see why later), which can complicate diagnosis and treatment. In general, however, reversible airway obstruction produces asthma's four hallmark symptoms:

- cough, which may be the main or only symptom in mild asthma;
- wheeze: a whistling, sighing sound caused when air passes through a narrow tube; asthmatic wheeze tends to be worse in the morning,

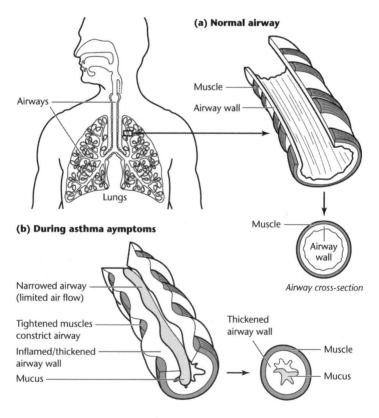

Figure 1.3 Normal (a) and asthmatic (b) airways

when the airways are naturally narrower (see pp. 26 and 60), during exercise or in cold air;

- shortness of, or gasping for, breath – night-time breathlessness may be a particularly reliable indicator of asthma in adults from early middle age onwards;
- chest tightness: some people describe this as a band around their chest. In my case, I felt as if I was lying under a paving slab.

Bronchial hyper-responsiveness – another hallmark of asthma we'll encounter throughout the book – refers to the tendency of asthmatic airways to narrow excessively and too readily when exposed to numerous non-allergic triggers, such as cold air, fog, perfume and tobacco smoke. Everyone's airways narrow in a smoky room to protect the lungs. However, in people with asthma, the narrowing is much more marked and occurs when you are exposed to much lower levels of the trigger than people with healthy lungs. Indeed, people with asthma tend to show increased bronchial hyper-responsiveness even before symptoms emerge. And those patients with more severe bronchial hyper-responsiveness tend to endure worse asthma symptoms than people with less reactive airways.

Asthma's sex divide

During childhood, boys are more likely to develop asthma than girls. The sex difference then switches. Middle-aged women are more likely to develop asthma than men of the same age. However, the difference between the sexes then declines again. The Lung and Asthma Information Agency points out that one study found that around 5 per cent of older men and 2 per cent of older women have asthma. But there are too few studies to know definitely whether elderly men are more likely to have asthma than women or vice versa. As you might expect, the pattern of bronchial hyper-responsiveness parallels the sex divide in asthma. The airways of boys are more responsive than those of girls, adult women are more responsive than men, and older men show broadly the same degree of responsiveness as older women.

A variable disease

No two asthma patients show exactly the same pattern of symptoms or endure the same impact on their life, health and well-being. And the severity of asthma and the frequency of attacks often varies over time in the same person. The variation in symptoms is especially marked in young children and older adults.

Occasionally people endure all four symptoms all the time. Some people experience debilitating attacks of all four symptoms, but only occasionally. Others endure just a troublesome cough and only during the night. Others find that they're symptom-free until they take part in certain activities – such as at work or during exercise.

Not surprisingly, this variation can complicate diagnosis, especially as the person may seem well and have near normal lung function between attacks. To complicate matters further, several diseases cause symptoms similar to asthma (see Chapter 5). So, doctors cannot diagnose asthma definitively using symptoms alone.

For instance, some asthmatics never wheeze audibly, and not everyone who wheezes suffers from asthma. Any disease that narrows the airways can cause wheeze:

- People with asthma and COPD tend to wheeze when they exhale.
- In some diseases – such as cancer in the trachea – wheeze tends to occur when the person breathes in.
- People develop reversible airway obstruction – and therefore wheeze and cough – when they contract a viral or bacterial lung infection.

This overlap in symptoms between asthma and other diseases further complicates diagnosis – especially as people may suffer from more than one disease.

Coughing up blood

If you cough up blood (the medical term is haemoptysis), you should seek medical attention as soon as possible. Haemoptysis may be the first sign of lung cancer and may allow doctors to detect the tumour when it remains small enough for surgery to cure. Several other serious diseases can cause haemoptysis, including tuberculosis and some other lung infections, chronic bronchitis and pulmonary oedema (fluid in the lungs).

When to seek urgent medical help

Never underestimate the severity of an asthma attack. During some severe asthma attacks, the airways become completely blocked and the person can suffocate, a potentially fatal condition called *status asthmaticus*. Ironically, people with the most severe asthma often have the worst perception of their symptoms' intensity. So, you should phone 999 immediately if you have any of the symptoms in the box below.

But try not to panic. Deaths from asthma are rare and effective prompt treatment prevents most fatalities. Furthermore, asthma attacks rarely strike out of the blue – although it can appear that way. Severe asthma attacks usually (but not always) develop over between 6 and 48 hours. This means that remaining alert to changes in your symptoms and regularly measuring your peak flow (see Chapter 5) might allow you to detect the decline and use your medication to prevent a serious attack. As we'll see in Chapter 6, you and your doctor should agree a self-management plan to deal with changes in symptom severity. A frank chat with your doctor or asthma nurse should help you keep your fears in perspective.

When to call 999

You (or someone around you) should call 999 if:

- you feel your bronchodilator (reliever) is not really helping your symptoms;
- the wheeze, cough or chest tightness is severe and constant. Wheeze may be especially loud or, ironically, absent in very severe asthma, when there is insufficient airflow to produce the sound. Medical schools traditionally warned doctors to 'beware of the silent chest';
- you are too breathless to speak, or talk in words rather than sentences;
- your pulse is racing;
- you feel agitated or restless;
- you feel drowsy or confused;
- your lips or fingernails look blue.

Some people hunch forward during a severe attack, which offers a further clue.

Suffering a severe asthma attack is terrifying and debilitating. One severe asthma attack left me unable to pick up the phone to call for an ambulance, let alone have a conversation. So, it's worth letting your partner, carer or colleagues know how to recognize the symptoms of a severe attack, and when to call 999. You could photocopy the box above and pin it to a notice board at home or work.

What goes wrong in asthma?

After a typhoon devastated the Pacific island of Tokelau, the authorities evacuated some children to New Zealand. Researchers discovered that asthma was just as common among the evacuated children as among kids born in New Zealand. However, asthma was much less common among children who remained on Tokelau than in the ex-pats or those born in New Zealand. Similarly, asthma and other allergic diseases became more common in people who moved from the former East to West Germany during the 1990s.

Clearly, environmental factors contribute to asthma. However, not everyone exposed to any particular environmental trigger develops asthma. For example, around 2 per cent of people develop asthma during their first year of working with animals. So, 49 in every 50 people working with animals don't develop asthma.

The pattern of genes we inherit helps determine whether or not we develop asthma when exposed to a potential trigger. Essentially, asthma arises when this combination of environmental factors and genes results in the airways' defences becoming 'over-protective'.

Protective airways

Every breath we take carries millions of potentially harmful micro-organisms (viruses, bacteria and fungi), potential allergens (immune triggers such as pollen or cat hair) and irritants (for example, tobacco smoke and pollutants) deep into our lungs. After all, micro-organisms are everywhere. Each square centimetre of human skin harbours around 10 million bacteria, *New Scientist* reported. Indeed, we breathe in about two heaped tablespoons of dust, pollen, mould, smoke, carbon, tar, rubber, metals and bacteria each day, along with countless chemicals.

To protect our delicate respiratory system and our bodies generally, our lungs evolved several lines of defence. For example, goblet cells lining the bronchi produce sticky mucus, which traps particles and pathogens. Tiny 'hairs' – called cilia – on the outside of cells lining the airways waft the mucus from the airways into your mouth. After you swallow the mucus, enzymes in your gut and acid in your stomach destroy the infection or particle. Coughing also removes mucus, particles and pathogens.

Poorly controlled asthma can damage this 'mucociliary escalator', which may leave you more vulnerable to lung infections. In turn, these infections can trigger an asthma attack. Smoking also damages the mucociliary escalator, one of the links between passive and active smoking and lung diseases such as asthma and COPD.

Second, a ring of muscle surrounds each airway. When this ring of muscle contracts, it squeezes and narrows the airway. This 'broncho-constriction' prevents harmful particles from penetrating deep into the lungs and reaching and potentially damaging the delicate alveoli. Smoking, for example, triggers bronchoconstriction in people without asthma. However, bronchial hyper-responsiveness (see above) means that people with asthma react excessively to non-allergic triggers such as smoking, cold air and pollution.

Inflammation offers a further line of defence in the airways and elsewhere in your body. During inflammation, blood vessels supplying the injured or infected area swell (dilate) and become leaky, which produces several characteristic changes:

- The increased blood flow makes the inflamed areas look red and feel warm.
- The movement of fluid from leaky blood vessels into the surrounding inflamed tissues causes swelling.
- The leaky vessels allow white blood cells and other components of the immune system to move into the damaged or infected tissue. For example, one type of white blood cell (phagocytes) engulfs and destroys invading micro-organisms and particles.
- The fluid contains chemicals that trigger pain, which stops you moving the injured area, so helping to prevent further damage.

So, inflammation starts healing. However, you can have too much of a good thing.

Too much of a good thing . . .

Inflammation usually subsides as an injury heals or the immune system eradicates an infection. Similarly, asthmatic symptoms resolve as the inflammation subsides, spontaneously or after treatment. However, while most lung infections last only a few days, sensitive people may be exposed to their asthma triggers continually (such as house dust mites) or for protracted periods (pollen, for instance). This means that people with asthma develop long-lasting (chronic) inflammation.

Over time, chronic inflammation alters the airway's structure – a process called remodelling. For example, chronic inflammation can destroy the delicate cilia and increase the number of goblet cells. The resulting rise in mucus production can create 'plugs' that block the airways. The damage to the mucociliary escalator makes these plugs difficult to remove.

Chronic inflammation also scars and thickens the airway walls. The more severe the asthma, the thicker the airway wall becomes. Indeed, Elias remarked, compared to people without asthma, the thickness of the airway wall increases by between 50 and 300 per cent in people who die from asthma. Even in non-fatal asthma, wall thickness can increase by between 10 and 100 per cent. As a result, remodelling permanently reduces the diameter of the airways in people with asthma, which makes a severe attack more likely. Furthermore, these changes tend to be irreversible. So, while doctors generally regard asthmatic airway obstruction as reversible, remodelling can cause at least partially irreversible symptoms.

Two main types of asthma

Doctors recognize several asthma subtypes that may differ in cause, symptoms, response to treatment and long-term outcome. Broadly, doctors split asthma into two types. First, in many people – especially children – asthma arises from an allergy (allergic asthma). However, in many adults, asthmatic inflammation seems to arise without an allergic reaction – so-called 'intrinsic' asthma. Some other forms of asthma – such as nocturnal and exercise-induced symptoms – overlap with these two main types (see Chapter 2).

Atopic (allergic) asthma

Allergic asthma's causes are very complex and scientists still haven't worked out all the details. Essentially, however, allergic triggers (allergens) travel deep into the lungs and come to rest on the thin layer of cells that lines the airways. This cell layer – called the respiratory epithelium – forms a barrier that stops disease-causing bacteria, viruses, fungi and other airborne hazards from entering the body. The respiratory epithelium also keeps the airways moist and contains mucus-producing goblet cells, which, as mentioned earlier, are an important defence against pathogens.

Specialist 'dendritic' cells in the respiratory epithelium engulf and ingest allergens and invading micro-organisms. Enzymes inside the dendritic cell degrade proteins in the allergen or pathogen into small fragments, called peptides. (Enzymes are specialized proteins that control biochemical reactions.) Dendritic cells then move to the local lymph nodes. These glands produce lymph, a liquid that bathes cells, and certain white blood cells that target the peptide fragments. (The same mechanism causes lymph nodes around your neck to swell during an infection. That's why a doctor feels your glands when you're unwell.)

Red, white and other blood cells

Blood contains many different types of cell. Red blood cells (erythrocytes) carry oxygen from your lungs to your tissues. Platelets help your blood clot. And white blood cells fight infections. For instance, lymph nodes produce several members of a family of white blood cells called T-lymphocytes. Each of the several T cell types has a specialized function:

- Memory T-lymphocytes help the body respond rapidly to microorganisms that it's encountered before.
- Cytotoxic T cells destroy the invading pathogen.
- T suppressor cells inhibit the immune response, helping to prevent it from raging out of control and destroying healthy tissue.

We're interested in another member of this family: T-helper cells (Th cells). Dendritic cells bind to and activate Th cells. In turn, Th cells release chemicals (cytokines) that stimulate another group of white blood cells (B cells), which form in the bone marrow.

B cells have two main actions. First, B cells produce antibodies, which allow your body to remember and respond rapidly to allergens and pathogens you have encountered before. The human immune system contains hundreds of millions of different B cells, each of which recognizes a different antigen or pathogen. Second, B cells activate other defensive white blood cells. (See Figure 1.4.)

Essentially, your immune system produces two main types of Th cells:

- Th_1 cells help the immune system tackle some bacteria and certain viruses.
- Th_2 lymphocytes evolved to protect against certain parasitic infections, especially gastrointestinal worms.

Many common allergens – such as house dust mites, pollen, animal dander (dead skin and fur) and fungal spores – contain proteases. These enzymes damage the respiratory epithelium, which activates the Th_2 response.

The first time you encounter an allergen you generally do not experience any symptoms. However, your immune system is 'primed'

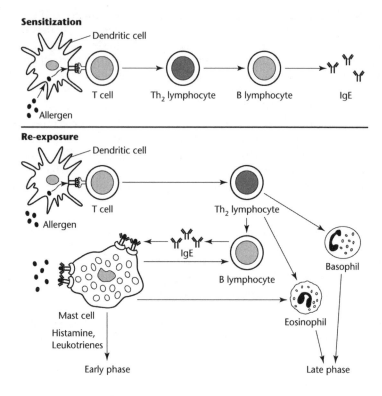

Figure 1.4 The immune response

(sensitized). So, when you next encounter the allergen, you quickly produce large amounts of antibodies.

This rapid response helps the immune system tackle infections. The first time you encounter a pathogen – such as chickenpox or a flu strain – you can suffer unpleasant, even serious, symptoms. However, sensitization means that your immune system swings into action and eradicates the infection much more quickly when you next encounter the pathogen, in many cases before you develop symptoms. This is, essentially, the same process as vaccination. The jab primes your immune system.

In allergies, however, this 'priming' means that the immune system produces symptoms when sensitive patients encounter triggers that most people find innocuous, such as cat or dog hair or grass pollen. In asthma, the reaction causes allergic symptoms in the lungs. In rhinitis and eczema, symptoms develop in the nose and skin respectively.

Introducing antibodies

B cells produce five families of antibody (called IgA, IgD, IgE, IgG and IgM), each of which controls a different aspect of the immune response. For instance, we evolved immunoglobulin E (IgE) to tackle certain parasites, including tapeworms. However, people with asthma triggered by cat dander produce IgE specific for cat dander. Those asthmatics sensitive to grass pollen produce IgE specific for grass pollen.

Immune changes with age

Several aspects of the immune response change with advancing age. For example, the T cell response seems to be less active in elderly adults compared to younger people. In particular, memory T-lymphocytes seem to become less responsive. This may contribute to allergies' declining importance as an asthmatic trigger in adults compared to children. Interestingly, women usually have lower levels of total and allergen-specific IgE than men. This observation ties in with the typical patient with intrinsic asthma: a middle-aged woman.

In general, IgE does not cross-react between allergens. So, IgE for cat dander won't trigger an allergic response when you encounter grass pollen. But there are occasional exceptions. For example, some pollens (such as birch) contain proteins that have a very similar structure to those in other plants, including apples, oranges, potatoes and tomatoes. This means that someone who produces IgE to, say, birch pollen may also develop allergic symptoms when peeling potatoes. Doctors call these proteins 'pan-allergens'.

IgE binds to yet another type of white blood cell, called mast cells. The great German scientist Paul Ehrlich noted during the 1870s that mast cells accumulate in inflamed areas. Ehrlich believed that the cells helped meet the inflamed tissue's increased nutritional requirements. So, he called them 'mast' cells – the German for 'fattening' or 'suckling'.

But we now know that mast cells are central to the immune response. IgE's binding triggers the release of mast cells' stores of inflammatory mediators, of which histamine is the best known. When IgE binds, mast cells also freshly make several other mediators that promote inflammation. Meanwhile, IgE also binds to basophils, another type of white blood cell, which trigger the release of yet more inflammatory mediators.

Some mediators released by mast cells and basophils attract other types of white blood cells into the inflamed tissue. These late-arriving cells add still more mediators into the cocktail, which help maintain the inflammation. The late-arriving cells also release enzymes and other chemicals that start breaking down inflamed tissue. This attack on inflamed tissue helps destroy invading pathogens, but also contributes to airway remodelling in asthma.

One type of late-arriving white blood cell, the eosinophil, seems to be especially important in asthma. Mediators and other chemicals released by eosinophils promote airway obstruction, contribute to remodelling and increase bronchial hyper-responsiveness in asthma. Indeed, eosinophils are present in the airway wall across all severities of asthma, from mild to life-threatening, and seem to be one of the key cells driving asthma.

The early and late allergic reactions

This immune reaction creates two 'peaks' in allergic symptoms. The early response in people with allergic asthma (driven, predominantly, by mast cells) reaches a peak after about 20 minutes of exposure to the allergen. Eosinophils and other late-arriving white blood cells usually take several hours to reach significant numbers in the inflamed tissue. As a result, allergic symptoms may re-emerge later, usually between 6 and 12 hours after the first exposure to the allergen. This is the so-called 'late-phase reaction'.

Uncontrolled inflammation could spread from the site of exposure and destroy the surrounding healthy tissue. So, the body evolved 'anti-inflammatory' mechanisms. For example, some mediators damp down the inflammation, limiting the immune response to damaged or infected tissue. Low levels of these mediators – as well as high levels of pro-inflammatory chemicals – can contribute to COPD and asthma. Furthermore, as mentioned on page 15, T suppressor cells help limit any collateral damage to healthy tissue during an inflammatory reaction. These mechanisms mean that the inflammation gradually subsides once your exposure to the allergen ends or the infection resolves.

Intrinsic asthma

Allergic (sometimes called extrinsic) asthma generally occurs in younger people, depends on IgE and tends to emerge in people whose immune system is highly sensitive to a particular allergen. In contrast, intrinsic asthma tends to occur in older people, doesn't involve IgE and shows a strong relationship with several non-allergic triggers, including certain respiratory infections, chronic sinusitis and recurrent bronchitis. Virchow notes that in one study, recurrent bronchitis preceded 17 per cent of cases of intrinsic asthma. Furthermore, 32 per cent of patients reported suffering a flu-like infection, while 51 per cent had chronic sinusitis and nasal polyps (Chapter 4). Typically, these conditions developed into persistent cough and then airway obstruction and wheeze.

Your age when symptoms first emerged may offer a clue as to whether you suffer from intrinsic or extrinsic asthma. Intrinsic asthma usually emerges in people aged between 40 and 50 years. Indeed, some doctors suggest regarding asthma that emerges before the age of 30 years as allergic until proven otherwise. On the other hand, they suggest considering asthma that emerges after the age of 40 years as intrinsic until proven otherwise. Sex offers another clue: three adult women suffer from intrinsic asthma for every two men with the disease. In part, this sex difference may reflect the impact of female hormones, an issue we'll return to later.

Children with allergic asthma often report that their siblings have allergic rhinitis (an allergy affecting the nose – hay fever is the best-known example), allergic asthma or allergic eczema (an allergic skin rash). With allergies' declining importance as a cause of asthma, such reports become less common in people whose asthma symptoms begin in later life. Nevertheless, many people with adult-onset (and, therefore, supposedly intrinsic) asthma report that they or another member of their family or both suffer from allergic diseases. Indeed, Virchow comments that one study showed that levels of IgE to house dust mite rose – remember, increased IgE is supposedly the hallmark of allergic asthma – before men with an average age of 64 years started wheezing. In another study, 21 per cent of people with 'intrinsic asthma' showed elevated levels of IgE. However, as we'll see in Chapter 5, showing IgE circulating in your blood doesn't necessarily mean that the immune response triggered by the allergen was sufficient to cause asthmatic symptoms. And in some people both mechanisms may play a role. If you think this sounds confusing – you're right! No clear picture emerges.

In the end, however, persistent inflammation drives intrinsic and allergic asthma. In addition, the lungs show similar changes – including reversible airway obstruction, exercise-induced symptoms, variations in lung function over the course of the day and raised levels of eosinophils – whether the asthma is intrinsic or allergic. So, the distinction between allergic and intrinsic asthma usually has little influence on diagnosis or treatment. Nevertheless, if you suffer from allergic asthma, identifying the cause may help you avoid the trigger.

Genes and asthma

Asthma, especially allergic asthma, runs strongly in families. Indeed, genetic factors may account for up to 60 per cent of the risk of developing asthma, according to Moffat and co-workers. Doctors describe the 30 to 40 per cent of the population with a tendency to produce excessive levels of IgE, especially when inherited, as 'atopic'. Allergic rhinitis (which includes hay fever) and the allergic forms of asthma and eczema are the 'atopic' diseases.

Researchers believe that more than 100 genes increase the risk of developing allergy and asthma. Rather than one gene strongly influencing the risk of developing asthma and allergies, several genes, each of which produces a moderate effect, seem to interact. Some of these genes increase the risk of asthma irrespective of age. A gene is an instruction that tells the cell to make a particular protein. For example, some of the age-independent genes code for proteins that 'report' damage to the airway epithelium to the immune system. These 'reports' activate inflammation driven by Th_2 cells, Moffat and co-workers remark.

Other genes linked to asthma throughout life produce proteins that down-regulate the immune system. In other words, the genes code for a protein that puts a brake on the airway inflammation. If the gene encodes an abnormal version of this protein, the inflammation will be poorly controlled. Finally, some genes determine the extent of airway remodelling whether you're 6 or 60 years old.

Other genes seem to influence the risk of developing asthma during childhood but not as an adult, or vice versa. Your cells contain 23 pairs of chromosomes. You inherited one copy of the chromosome in each pair from your mother, the other from your father. This means that you have 46 chromosomes. (Down's syndrome and certain other genetic diseases are exceptions to this rule. Down's Syndrome, for example, arises when the child inherits an additional copy of part or all of chromosome 21 during conception.)

One study looked for genes linked to asthma across all 23 pairs of chromosomes. Moffat and colleagues found a particularly strong link between a region on chromosome 17 and asthma in children. In contrast, a region on chromosome 6 exerted an important influence on the risk of adult-onset asthma and seemed to code for a protein that influences the immune response provoked by bacterial or other non-atopic (non-allergic) triggers. These genetic variations underscore, once again, that in some cases asthma in children and adults may be very different diseases, despite the superficial similarity in symptoms.

Human DNA has contained most – if not all – of the genes linked to asthma for thousands – if not millions – of years. But the number of cases of allergic asthma and other atopic diseases rose dramatically in children during the twentieth century. The Lung and Asthma Information Agency estimates that the number of children with asthma increased by about half between the early 1970s and the mid 1980s. (The agency also notes that there are too few studies to assess whether the number of adults with asthma increased.) Moreover, the number of people with allergic eczema increased between two- and three-fold in the last 30 years of the twentieth century.

Alterations in our genetic code could not account for the rapid rise in these allergic diseases. In any case, as mentioned at the start of this chapter, the interaction between genes and environment determines your risk of developing asthma. Against this background, the 'hygiene hypothesis' (see the box below) helps explain the marked rise in asthma and other atopic diseases.

The 'hygiene hypothesis'

Whether an immature Th cell becomes a Th_1 or Th_2 lymphocyte depends on the hazards in the environment. Many bacterial infections 'programme' the immune system to produce Th_1 cells. Th_2 cells protect against certain parasites and several other infections. During the twentieth century, improved sanitation, better nutrition and vaccinations reduced the risk of infections. So, 'idling' Th_2 cells started responding to allergens.

This means that the bacteria, viruses and other pathogens that you encounter in early life seem to influence your risk of going on to develop asthma. For example, most studies (although not all) suggest that infections with parasitic worms protect against asthma and other allergies. The Th_2 cells target the parasite rather than the lung. Furthermore, the respiratory syncytial virus (RSV) causes the common cold in adults and bronchiolitis (inflammation of the bronchioles) in children. RSV infections augment Th_2 responses, and therefore seem to be a risk factor for developing asthma later in life.

On the other hand, certain microbes boost the Th_1 response. So there are fewer Th_2 cells, which may reduce the risk of asthma. This probably partly explains why children with older brothers and sisters are less likely to be asthmatic than those without elder siblings. Younger children are more likely to catch a childhood infection, and therefore have fewer Th_2 cells and a lower risk of asthma.

In other words, the person's particular pattern of exposure to allergens and microbes in early childhood may programme the immune system to 'favour' a particular Th pattern and therefore influence the risk of developing allergic asthma. As our homes and environment became cleaner, as our nutrition improved and as vaccinations prevented many of the diseases most feared by our parents and grandparents, the patterns of exposure to pathogens changed. These changes contributed to the rise in asthma and, probably, the other atopic diseases during the twentieth century. However, other factors – including alterations in diet – probably also contributed to the changing risk of allergies.

Studying asthma's genetics helps researchers understand the causes of the disease and may lead to new treatments. However currently, doctors cannot look at your genetic code and determine your risk of developing asthma. They can't predict the course of your asthma, your response to treatment or the severity of your symptoms after analysing your genetic code and risk factors.

Nevertheless, in the future doctors may be able to scan a person's genetic code, characterize a person's chance of developing asthma, predict the severity and ascertain which treatment will be the most effective and least likely to cause side effects. We have only just scratched the surface of the potential offered by genetic studies into asthma.

2

Types of asthma

Asthma isn't really a single disease. It's an umbrella term, covering various patterns of symptoms and a multitude of causes. This chapter looks at some of the common types of asthma, which may overlap.

You should discuss your particular pattern of symptoms with your doctor or asthma nurse to help optimize your treatment. For example, from time to time most people with asthma experience symptoms when they exercise particularly heavily or during the occasional night. However, *regularly* suffering exercise-induced and nocturnal symptoms may indicate that your asthma is poorly controlled and so your dose of anti-inflammatory (preventer) might need to rise (see Chapter 6). On the other hand, some people experience symptoms *only* following exercise or during the night. As we'll see, treatment may differ in each case.

Severe asthma

Between 5 and 10 per cent of asthmatics suffer severe symptoms – that's around half a million British people, according to Asthma UK. While definitions vary, essentially severe symptoms remain poorly controlled despite repeated courses of standard drugs (usually including high doses of inhaled corticosteroid and oral steroids) and despite people sticking to their treatment.

Severe asthma can take several forms. Some people suffer asthma symptoms almost continually, despite taking steroids and other anti-inflammatory medications (see Chapter 6). Other patients with 'brittle asthma' endure severe attacks but have normal lung function and don't experience marked symptoms in between. Others endure mild asthma that occasionally flares into a severe attack, despite taking their medication.

Several factors can contribute to severe asthma:

- Continual or repeated exposure to an allergen (such as house dust mite, cockroach or some fungi such as *Alternaria*) can lead to severe asthma.
- Airway remodelling can also contribute to severe asthma, in which

case symptoms usually worsen gradually, often over several years. (Nevertheless, some adults show a relatively rapid decline in lung function over ten years or less, especially if they developed asthma for the first time aged over 60 years.)

- Asthma that persists from childhood tends to be more severe than asthma that first emerges in adults. For instance, Ségala and colleagues found that 31 per cent of adult asthmatics reporting no childhood asthma experienced less than one attack per month. In contrast, just 15 per cent of patients who recalled having asthma as a child suffered less than one exacerbation a month.
- Respiratory infections – such as the bacteria *Mycoplasma pneumoniae* and *Chlamydophila pneumoniae* – commonly trigger severe asthma in adults.
- More than 80 per cent of people with severe asthma have sinusitis: inflammation of the sinuses in the face (see page 39). It's not clear whether sinusitis causes severe asthma, whether sinusitis and asthma arise from the same underlying inflammation, or both.
- Smoking increases the frequency and severity of symptoms and exacerbations, and hastens the decline in lung function. So do all you can to quit (Chapter 7). However, severe asthma also develops in lifelong non-smokers.
- Around three-quarters of people with severe asthma are overweight or obese. Chapter 7 offers some tips to help you shed weight.

As this diversity suggests, you and your doctor will need to examine the details of your management, asthma patterns and lifestyle to determine your most appropriate treatment.

Recalcitrant asthma

Often doctors and patients lump recalcitrant and severe asthma together. However, they're different: 'recalcitrant asthma' refers to symptoms that fail to respond adequately to treatment. As you may expect, many people with recalcitrant asthma suffer severe symptoms. However, mild symptoms might not respond fully to treatment, while some cases of severe life-threatening asthma improve quickly once treatment begins.

Recalcitrant asthma arises from several causes:

- The doctor may misdiagnose asthma. Several diseases – such as COPD, congestive heart failure and vocal cord dysfunction – can mimic asthma's symptoms. Treatments for asthma often aren't effective in these other conditions. Indeed, they can make matters worse.

Unfortunately, diagnosing asthma can prove especially difficult in older people or those with more than one ailment. So, if your asthma treatment doesn't seem to be working, you could ask your doctor to investigate whether another condition could be responsible.

- Recalcitrant symptoms can emerge if you and your doctor don't adequately control a factor that increases asthma severity – such as indoor allergens, smoking, sinusitis or gastro-oesophageal reflux disease (GORD). People with GORD regurgitate small amounts of stomach acid into their mouth. Some of this can seep into the trachea and lungs, exacerbating the severity of their asthma (see Chapter 3). Tackling any exacerbating factors can enhance the response to anti-asthma medicines.
- Doctors and asthma nurses don't always treat asthma aggressively enough. Some doctors may, for example, not increase the steroid dose or suggest an additional treatment because they worry about side effects. (The principle 'first do no harm' is one of medicine's most important ethical and intellectual foundations.) There are now guidelines for asthma control, which offer doctors clear advice on when to increase treatment and the most appropriate drug (see Chapter 6).
- Patients fail to take their medication as advised by the doctor or asthma nurse – so-called poor 'compliance', 'adherence' or 'concordance'. Some people may deliberately not take their medicines because they feel they don't need the drug or because they worry about side effects. This book, and a full and frank discussion of the risks and benefits with your GP or asthma nurse, should resolve concerns about the efficacy or safety of your treatment (see Chapter 3).
- Remodelling and other severe complications of asthma can lead to recalcitrant symptoms as the obstruction becomes 'fixed' and less responsive to treatment. Alternatively, the inflammation may simply be too severe for steroids to tackle effectively.
- Some people show a markedly impaired response to steroids, the mainstay of treatment for asthmatic inflammation. As Adcock and Barnes note, researchers are only beginning to unravel the complex causes of steroid resistance. However, some people (perhaps because of their genetic code) produce too few or insensitive steroid receptors (receptors bind the steroid, which starts a chain of events that ends with the anti-inflammatory action – see Chapter 6). In other cases, the chain of events inside the cell through which steroids reduce inflammation seems to be dysfunctional.

Fortunately, research is beginning to yield new treatments for severe asthma. For example, omalizumab (see Chapter 6) offers an option for adults and adolescents with severe, persistent and unstable allergic asthma.

Nocturnal asthma: a wake-up call

Among other important actions, sleep helps consolidate memories and learning, protected our ancestors from attack by predators, and aids mental and physical recuperation. Given its biological importance, it's not surprising that sleep disturbances potentially cause considerable distress. However, according to a survey carried out by Asthma UK, 61 per cent of asthmatics say that respiratory symptoms stop them from getting a good night's sleep, which can leave the person tired, irritable and sleepy the next day. Tired people are also more likely to have accidents and their performance at work or college can suffer.

As the survey shows, around 60 per cent of people with asthma find that wheezing and other symptoms are worse at night and in the early morning – so-called nocturnal asthma. Some people experience symptoms only at night. Three main changes contribute to this pattern:

- Nocturnal asthma symptoms reflect the natural variation in the diameter of the bronchi over the course of the day. Even in healthy people, changes in the airway diameter mean that lung function peaks around 4 p.m. and reaches a nadir around 4 a.m. However, the difference between peak and trough lung function is much greater in asthma patients than in people with healthy lungs.
- Inflammation seems to worsen during the night in people with nocturnal asthma more than in people with asthma of similar severity who do not wake at night wheezing or breathless. For example, levels of some mediators produced by the body to bolster or reduce inflammation vary over the course of the day.
- Many people with asthma experience their most severe chest tightness and wheezing when they get up in the morning. This seems to reflect the combination of narrow bronchi, increased physical activity and worse inflammation.

Nocturnal asthma remains under-diagnosed, partly because some asthmatics feel that the disturbed nights are an inevitable part of the disease. Other people seem to feel that changes in sleep patterns are part of ageing. Certainly, around half of elderly people report insomnia and poor sleep quality. Nevertheless, you should not dismiss a disturbed night's sleep as simply part of growing older. Nocturnal symptoms should be a wake-up call for you to see your doctor or asthma nurse. Waking at night wheezing or breathless is one of the strongest indicators that your asthma is poorly controlled.

Exercise-induced asthma

Healers knew that exercise could induce asthma more than 1,800 years ago. Today, doctors recognize that exercise can trigger symptoms in 80 to 90 per cent of people with asthma. Some people experience asthma symptoms *only* when they exercise. Nevertheless, exercise-induced symptoms are not an excuse to become a couch potato. Indeed, Sinha and David note, 29 per cent of elite athletes show exercise-induced bronchoconstriction. Furthermore, exercise helps alleviate asthma (by improving lung function) and helps counter some other risk factors linked to the disease, such as obesity.

Elaine's exercise-induced asthma

Her school asked Elaine, a 28-year-old teaching assistant, to help with the netball club and PE classes. She'd not really exercised since leaving school but agreed, especially as it would help her lose the extra weight she'd put on since giving birth to her daughter four years before. However, about ten minutes into the class, breathlessness forced Elaine to the sidelines. Elaine thought she was just unfit. But every time she took part or tried to jog around the park to boost her fitness, she had to stop every five or ten minutes to catch her breath, and kept coughing and wheezing. She didn't smoke and wondered if she was anaemic. But her doctor suspected exercise-induced asthma. Taking a short-acting bronchodilator 15 minutes before exercise allowed Elaine to take an active part in the class and club. She's been jogging regularly and is training towards taking part in the local half-marathon to raise funds for the school.

So why do some people experience exercise-related bronchoconstriction? When you exercise, your muscles demand more oxygen. In response, your heart beats more quickly, your respiration rate rises and your bronchi dilate to let more air into the lungs. In healthy people, bronchi remain open throughout exercise. But in people with exercise-induced asthma, the drier and cooler air you inhale during exercise triggers the bronchi to narrow, usually between five and 15 minutes after you start working out.

As your respiration rate rises, you are less able to humidify and warm the increased amount of air you breathe in. In sensitive patients, especially in people with pre-existing inflammation, increased evaporation of water from the lungs triggers the release of mediators from mast cells (including histamine and leukotrienes). The resulting bronchoconstriction can cause chest pain, breathlessness, cough and wheeze during or after exercise. Cold air increases the dehydration and exacerbates the airway narrowing.

So you may have exercise-induced bronchospasm if you experience one or more of the following between five and 15 minutes after starting to work out:

- Shortness of breath or chest tightness.
- You find your exercise endurance unexpectedly declines or doesn't improve when you increase your workouts.
- You cough or wheeze.

Some patients with exercise-induced asthma also suffer upset stomachs or a sore throat.

The timing of symptoms is critical. Symptoms that emerge during the first five minutes of a workout do not usually indicate exercise-induced asthma, but may indicate poorly controlled asthma, lack of fitness or injury to the muscles in your chest wall. So see your doctor, who may suggest that you take an exercise tolerance test, for example, to differentiate wheezing due to asthma from other causes of shortness of breath on exertion. Heart failure, severe anaemia and obesity, which are often exacerbated by poor physical fitness, can all cause shortness of breath during exercise.

It's worth making the effort to identify the cause and to get fit. Ironically, physical fitness is one of the best ways to beat exercise-induced bronchoconstriction. As your physical fitness improves, you use less of your vital capacity to exercise at any particular level of activity. Fitness also reduces the cooling and drying effect of air, and therefore the severity of bronchoconstriction triggered by exercise. The box below offers some suggestions that should reduce the risk of suffering symptoms while you work out. In other words, there is no excuse not to exercise! After all, 67 athletes at the 1984 Olympic Games suffered from asthma. So talk to your doctor or nurse first and pick up those trainers.

Preventing exercise-induced asthma

- Increase your physical fitness. If you're a member of a gym, ask them to review your programme. If not, think about joining.
- Warm up for at least ten minutes before exercising.
- Cover your mouth and nose with a scarf or mask when exercising in cold weather.
- If possible, exercise in a warm environment with humidified air.
- Avoid allergens and pollution – so don't jog through the woods or fields, or exercise in front of an open window on a polluted city street.
- At the end of exercise, cool down or gradually reduce the exercise intensity.
- Wait at least two hours after eating before exercising.
- Choose the right exercise. Running is more likely to trigger asthma than cycling, for instance. Both are more likely to induce asthma than swimming. As cold air is a common trigger, many people with asthma find ski-ing, skating and other winter sports trigger their symptoms.
- Take a short-acting bronchodilator 15 minutes before and, if needed, during exercise. You could also try sodium cromoglicate and nedocromil (see Chapter 6), which prevent exercise-induced symptoms in between 70 and 85 per cent of patients. You can discuss these options with your doctor or asthma nurse.

Drug-induced asthma

Every time you take aspirin or ibuprofen, you're part of a medical tradition stretching back thousands of years. Plants evolved a chemical called salicylic acid as part of their defences against disease. But our ancestors soon learnt that consuming a preparation of plants containing salicylates alleviated pain, inflammation and fever. For example, the Ebers Papyrus, an Egyptian text written some 3,500 years ago, suggests using herbal painkillers that we now know contain salicylates. Greek and Roman healers employed salicylate-containing plants to alleviate rheumatism. Traditional British healers used willow bark, which is rich in salicylic acid, to relieve pain and fever. In 1763, Edward Stone, a vicar in the Oxfordshire village of Chipping Norton, found that a dram (about 1.8 g) of willow bark extract alleviated fever.

German scientists synthesized salicylic acid chemically in 1860. A chemical variation, acetylsalicylic acid, followed in 1899, and was marketed as Aspirin. Today, the chemical offspring of natural salicylates and acetylsalicylic acid – a group of drugs called non-steroidal anti-inflammatory drugs (NSAIDs), which includes ibuprofen, diclofenac and naproxen – are among the most widely prescribed medicines.

Yet familiarity shouldn't breed complacency. NSAIDs can cause serious, even life-threatening side effects, including gastrointestinal ulcers and bleeding (haemorrhage), strokes and asthma. Indeed, aspirin may precipitate an attack in up to a fifth of people with asthma. Kuna and colleagues report the case of a 48-year-old Polish man who was so sensitive to aspirin that he suffered an attack following sexual intercourse with his wife after she'd taken aspirin – although only when he didn't use a condom.

So people with asthma should not use NSAIDs – even creams or gels, and even if bought without a prescription (over the counter) from a pharmacy or supermarket – without speaking to a doctor, pharmacist or nurse first. The risk of developing asthma symptoms rises as the NSAID dose increases. Therefore, even if the health professional agrees, make sure you follow the dosing instructions, take the minimum amount that controls your pain or inflammation, and use the medicine for the shortest time you can. If you develop a rash or suffer physical side effects such as difficulty breathing, dyspepsia (indigestion) or abdominal pain, stop using the NSAID and seek medical advice as soon as possible.

You should always tell pharmacists that you suffer from asthma and let them know what other medications you are taking – including herbal treatments – when buying an over-the-counter painkiller or flu remedy. Pharmacists can offer you alternatives (such as paracetamol). Asthmatics also need to be careful of some herbal medicines – see Chapter 7. As we've seen, many plants contain salicylates. So make sure that the herbalist knows you suffer from asthma (even if you're not consulting for respiratory symptoms). And your doctor, nurse and pharmacist should know if you're taking herbal supplements.

Other medicines that can trigger asthma

Several other medicines potentially trigger asthma in sensitive people. For example, doctors prescribe drugs called beta-blockers for, among other conditions, some cases of dangerously high blood pressure (hypertension), some anxiety symptoms and glaucoma. (In glaucoma, pressure exerted by fluids inside the eye damages the nerves carrying signals from the light-sensitive retina at the back of the eye to the brain. Untreated glaucoma can lead to blindness.)

Beta-blockers cause airways to narrow. In healthy people taking beta-blockers, the narrowing isn't enough to cause respiratory symptoms. However, in people with asthma the narrowing may provoke an attack. Enough beta-blocker can even reach the bloodstream from eye drops used to treat glaucoma to trigger bronchoconstriction. Fortunately, doctors can usually find an alternative medication that will not provoke exacerbations.

Rory and the hot dog

Rory, a 31-year-old sales executive, has suffered from asthma since childhood. And he knows that aspirin makes his asthma worse. So he carefully avoids taking NSAIDs, always reads the side of the box of any painkiller or cold and flu remedy he buys, and tells the pharmacist about his aspirin sensitivity. However, at a recent football match he suffered a severe asthma attack that left him wheezing and breathless during the second half of the important game. He assumed the excitement was responsible – 'Just my luck,' he lamented to his friends. But the attack happened again at another game, and then at his children's school fireworks display. He realized that on all three occasions he'd eaten hot dogs. At his next routine appointment, he asked – rather hesitantly – whether he could be allergic to hot dogs. The nurse mentioned that some hot dogs contain preservatives or a colour that might trigger his aspirin-sensitive asthma. Rory now sticks to burgers.

Food additives

Food manufacturers may use salicylates as preservatives in certain foods, including some hot dogs, ice cream, sandwich spreads, soft drinks and so on. A wide range of other preservatives as well as several colours and antioxidants can trigger asthma in sensitive people. For example, the yellow dye tartrazine triggers symptoms in around half of people with aspirin-sensitive asthma. (These are not allergies: IgE isn't involved.)

Salicylates also occur naturally in some fruits and vegetables. So totally avoiding salicylates is impracticable. But if you are sensitive, try to avoid those foods that seem to evoke a strong reaction – and always read the label. (You may need to keep a food diary to discover any foods that provoke symptoms in you.) Table 2.1 shows some common additives associated with asthma in sensitive people.

Table 2.1: Examples of additives that may provoke asthma symptoms in some sensitive people

E102	Tartrazine
E104	Quinoline yellow
E110	Sunset yellow
E122	Carmoisine
E123	Amaranth
E132	Indigo carmine
E142	Green S
E160b	Annatto
E210–219	Benzoates
E223	Sodium metabisulphite
E320	Butylated hydroxyanisole (BHA)
E321	Butylated hydroxytoluene (BHT)

Infective asthma

Many people with asthma complain that colds 'go to their chest', take more than ten days to clear up and exacerbate their symptoms. Indeed, respiratory infections are another very common asthma trigger: viruses may contribute to 80 per cent of exacerbations in children and adults.

In some cases, the infection's effects can last a lifetime: alveoli multiply and bronchi grow especially rapidly during the first three to four years of life. Dharmage and co-workers note that serious lung infections during this critical time could cause permanent damage and undermine lung function that persists into adult life.

Pathogens and asthma

Certain micro-organisms are especially likely to cause or exacerbate asthma. For example, rhinovirus – a group of more than 100 viruses responsible for many cases of the common cold – causes nearly two-thirds of infections linked to asthma exacerbations. In adults, infection with the bacterium *Chlamydophila pneumoniae* increased the risk of developing asthma over the next six months seven-fold compared with other respiratory infections.

Unfortunately, several age-related changes mean that older people are especially prone to catching pneumonia and other lung infections. For example:

- The cough reflex does not trigger as readily in older people. And each cough may generate less force than in younger people, so you're less able to clear the infection.
- As we get older, cilia are less able to remove mucus from the airway.
- The nose and airway secrete less IgA (an antibody that protects against viruses) as we age.
- The airways of older people tend to collapse more readily than is typical in a younger person during shallow breathing (for example, because of pain, illness or after surgery) or when the person is bed-bound for a long time. This further hinders the lungs' ability to clear the infection.

Against this background, it is very important that older people and younger people with severe asthma or other lung diseases receive their annual flu jab (Chapter 7). Furthermore, you should monitor your peak flow especially carefully during lung infections and increase your treatment according to your self-management plan (Chapter 6), when appropriate.

3

Common asthma triggers

In 1981, the number of adults admitted to hospitals in Barcelona suffering from asthma rose dramatically, but only at certain times. After two years trying to track down the cause, doctors realized that soybean dust released into the atmosphere during loading and unloading at the city's docks triggered the outbreaks. As this shows, environmental factors can trigger asthma in sensitive people, but identifying the cause can prove difficult. You may need to examine possible triggers at home, at work (see Chapter 4) and at play.

Some triggers (such as infections and exercise) overlap with the types of asthma we considered in the previous chapter. In this chapter, we will look at some other common asthma triggers. Chapter 7 offers some practical suggestions about how you can reduce their impact.

Jack's new hobby

Jack, a 35-year-old local government accountant, rarely leaves his office during work hours. But Jack plays rugby and cricket for his local village sides and is relatively fit. He's never suffered from breathing or chest problems before, but recently started feeling breathless at home and is waking several nights a week, coughing. Jack sees his GP as he's concerned about heart disease. However, his doctor realizes that Jack's developed asthma and tries to track down any obvious causes before referring for allergy testing. Jack bought his daughter a rabbit for her eighth birthday around the time the symptoms started, but his work commitments mean that he rarely comes into contact with the pet. The only other change has been that Jack's restarted an old hobby: electronics. He's currently building a new computer. The symptoms, Jack now recalls, started a month or so after he started working on the computer. The GP suggests that the solder – a common trigger for occupational asthma – may be responsible. After taking a break from his hobby for a couple of weeks, Jack's symptoms improve.

Allergens

As we saw in Chapter 1, the immune system evolved to recognize and eradicate invading micro-organisms. In people with allergic asthma, an allergen (immune trigger) inappropriately triggers the immune defences. However, while the immune system clears an invading bacterium, allergic asthma arises from chronic inflammation. For example, in children and young adults, being sensitive on skin-prick tests (Chapter 5) to indoor allergens (such as house dust mite or cat and dog dander) and the fungus *Alternaria* increases the risk of developing asthma between three- and twenty-fold. Furthermore, Ségala and colleagues found that adults who had asthma in childhood were more likely than those who developed asthma as adults to be sensitive to allergens such as house dust mite, dog hair, and grass and tree pollens.

Pollen

Fewer than 100 of the more than a quarter of a million plant species worldwide that produce pollen trigger asthma or other allergies in humans. Unfortunately, the 100 includes some of the most common plants. In the UK, for example, grass, tree and nettle are the most common pollen allergens. However, a wide variety of other flora can trigger asthma and other allergies, including some relatively exotic ornamental plants, such as *Ficus benjamina* (weeping fig or Benjamin's fig) and mimosa. Not surprisingly, the allergen responsible for pollen-related asthma varies worldwide as the flora changes. For example, between 10 and 20 per cent of Americans suffer from ragweed allergy, which can cause hay fever and asthma. Indeed, three-quarters of Americans who are allergic to pollen are sensitive to ragweed.

You don't need to live next to a meadow or wood to suffer pollen-triggered asthma. Some pollens travel 20 km from their source. Scientists found ragweed pollen 400 miles out to sea and two miles high in the atmosphere. On the other hand, grass pollen deposits within three metres of the parent plant. But grass is everywhere, even in the centre of towns and cities. Just think how quickly grass colonizes an urban wasteland. This makes avoiding grass pollen difficult, if not impossible. Nevertheless, as mentioned in Chapter 7, you can take several steps to reduce your exposure.

Fungi

Fungi are remarkably diverse. Biologists have identified more than 70,000 fungal species. Thousands more probably await discovery. Indeed, some mycologists estimate that 1.5 million species of fungi may exist amid life on earth, each of which has its own niche. The moulds around damp windows, yeasts used in bread and beer-making, and dermatophytes that colonize skin, hair and nails are all fungi.

Many fungi potentially pose health problems. AIDS patients, for example, can die from opportunistic fungal infections. The yeast *Candida albicans* causes vaginal and oral thrush – the latter can be a problem with inhaled steroids (see Chapter 6) – while dermatophytes cause athlete's foot, ringworm and 'jock itch'. And several fungi can trigger asthma.

For example, the fungi *Cladosporium* and *Alternaria* grow on dead organic material (such as decaying leaves). Levels of spores from these fungi peak around harvest time and can trigger severe asthma attacks in some people working outside. Furthermore, around 400 species of mould make their homes indoors. Look at the corner of a window where water collects or in the bathroom of a poorly ventilated house. The dark stain could be a mould such as *Aspergillus* or *Penicillium*, both of which can trigger asthma in sensitized people.

Indeed, moulds can grow almost anywhere, provided there's enough moisture and oxygen – even inside our lungs. Fairs and colleagues grew *Aspergillus fumigatus* from the sputum of 63 per cent of asthma patients who produced IgE specific for the fungus, 31 per cent of non-sensitized asthmatics and 7 per cent of healthy people. However, unlike plants, moulds can't produce food from sunlight and air, so they decompose plant or animal matter for nourishment. While moulds don't – unlike plants – have a reproductive season, warmth and high humidity tends to encourage their growth. As a result, spore levels peak in warm humid weather and are particularly high in bathrooms, showers and kitchens.

House dust mites

It's an unpleasant thought, but your beds, soft toys and carpets are home to millions of microscopic creatures that feed on dead skin cells and other debris – the ubiquitous house dust mite. A gram of house dust may contain up to 5,000 mites.

House dust mites are most at home in bedding, soft furnishings and dusty corners where there is plenty of dead skin. So you probably spend eight hours each night lying among the two million mites in a typical bed mattress. Meanwhile, the mites use enzymes to digest your dead skin cells. The enzymes accumulate in the mites' faeces. When inhaled, the enzymes can trigger the reaction that leads to asthma.

Animals

The UK is home to some 10.3 million cats and 10.5 million dogs. In 2007, 26 per cent of households owned cats and 31 per cent owned dogs, according to the *Veterinary Record*. We also own numerous other pets including fish, birds, horses, reptiles and other more exotic species. Furthermore, many people work with animals, in food production, science laboratories, zoos and pet shops. Not surprisingly, asthma and allergies triggered by animals are common.

Animals can shed particles of dead skin and hair (dander) or feathers that can cause severe allergies in sensitive people. So people who keep pigeons, budgerigars or other birds can become sensitive to feathers and develop 'pigeon fancier's lung'. Some people also become allergic to a particular animal's urine.

If you're allergic to an exotic, laboratory or farm animal, it's probably easy to limit your exposure (although, as we'll see in the next chapter, people who develop occupational asthma might lose their job). Avoiding allergens from domestic animals is more difficult, especially as few families want to rehome their loved pets. In any case, cat dander can cling to floors, soft furnishings and even the walls, so allergen levels can remain high more than nine months after the animal's removal. Furthermore, cats and dogs spread dander as they roam the house. Allergies caused by cats and dogs tend to worsen during the winter, when the house is less well ventilated and pets spend more time indoors. However, you can reduce your exposure – see Chapter 7.

Food allergies

Many parents believe that food allergies cause or contribute to their child's asthma. However, 'true' food allergies (in other words, caused by IgE specific for a protein in food) are very rare. For example, around 13 per cent of adults complain that certain foods trigger symptoms, such as asthma or intestinal complaints. However, only between one in every 500 and 10,000 adults are truly allergic.

Nevertheless, even if IgE isn't responsible for your symptoms, you may be intolerant to preservatives or colours, for example. (We've already seen that some preservatives are chemically related to salicylates and may trigger symptoms in people with aspirin-sensitive asthma.) If you feel that food causes or exacerbates your symptoms, you should keep a diary and discuss undergoing a specific test for antibodies to suspected foods with your GP or asthma nurse. If this suggests that a food may contribute to your asthma, a dietician will help you exclude it from your diet to see if your symptoms improve. You may also undergo a 'provocation' test to see if reintroducing the food triggers symptoms.

But don't be tempted to exclude the food from your diet yourself (you could cut out some important nutrients). And don't be tempted by 'alternative' diagnostic tests for food sensitivity. Little, if any, scientific evidence supports their use.

Sex

In some people, emotional excitement or physical exertion during sex can trigger an asthma attack, so the tips on managing exercise-induced asthma may help. Using a bronchodilator before sex may help prevent you becoming breathless for the wrong reasons.

Occasionally, highly sensitive people with asthma suffer an attack if they kiss someone who has consumed a food or medicine (such as NSAIDs) that triggers their exacerbations. Allergic people can be exquisitely sensitive, sometimes reacting several hours after their partner ingested the food or drug and even after they've brushed their teeth. Indeed, people may excrete certain triggers in their saliva as long as 16 to 24 hours after their body has absorbed the food or medicine. Furthermore, a few people are allergic to chemicals in spermicides, lubricants, latex (used in some condoms) or semen. Once again, keeping a diary and informing your partner of any drugs or foods that exacerbate your asthma may help reduce the risk of exacerbations.

Diseases linked to asthma

Asthma is one of the most common diseases in the UK. So, not surprisingly, many people suffer from one or more ailments in addition to asthma. Many of these 'concurrent' diseases have no impact on asthma or its treatment. But in some cases the concurrent disease undermines asthma control:

- Some diseases – such as arthritis – may make using inhalers difficult. Changing the inhaler, using an aid or, in some cases, oral medications can overcome problems caused by poor mobility (see Chapter 6).
- As we've seen with NSAIDs and beta-blockers, some medicines used to treat the concurrent disease can exacerbate asthma. Fortunately, doctors can usually find an alternative.
- Some diseases directly increase the risk of developing asthma or suffering an exacerbation. The rest of this chapter looks at some common examples.

Hay fever

We tend to regard rhinitis – inflammation of the nose, such as in hay fever – and asthma as separate diseases. However, the respiratory tract is a continuous organ that begins in the nose and ends at the alveoli. In addition, in many people with both diseases, the same trigger (e.g. pollen) underlies allergic rhinitis and asthma. (We'll see a striking example of this when we look at the effect of weather on asthma.) Indeed, inflammation that begins in the nose can spread to the lungs (or vice versa), eventually spreading throughout the entire respiratory tract. So people with asthma often develop rhinitis and vice versa. For example, occupational rhinitis is up to three times more common than work-related asthma (Chapter 4). However, Rachiotis and co-workers reported that between 76 and 92 per cent of people with occupational asthma also suffer from rhinitis.

On the other hand, this intimate relationship means that treating rhinitis can improve asthma – and vice versa. For example, steroid nasal sprays that alleviate rhinitis can reduce bronchial hyper-responsiveness. So if you also suffer from hay fever or perennial rhinitis (non-seasonal symptoms caused by, for example, animal allergens or house dust mites) you should ask your nurse or GP to help you optimize treatment of your nasal symptoms.

Chronic sinusitis and polyps

Sinuses are small cavities behind your cheekbones, eyes and forehead, and on either side of the bridge of your nose. These cavities open into your nasal airways and help control the temperature and water content of the air that enters your lungs. (As we've seen, cold, dry air can trigger asthma symptoms.)

Sinusitis occurs when the sinuses become inflamed and swollen, often during a common cold, influenza or another infection. Exposure to allergens or irritants – including air pollution, tobacco smoke and chemicals such as pesticides, disinfectants and household detergents – can also trigger or exacerbate sinusitis.

Usually, mucus produced by your sinuses drains into your nose through small channels. Infections and inflammation can block these channels and mucus fills the sinus, causing pain, tender areas on the face, a blocked or runny nose, and, in some cases, a fever. On average, sinusitis takes about two and a half weeks to resolve. Chronic sinusitis, which lasts more than 12 weeks, increases an adult's risk of developing asthma.

In some cases, for reasons that doctors don't fully understand, tissues lining the sinuses can swell and expand into the nose, forming a polyp (Figure 3.1). Some polyps seem to grow after an infection. In others, allergies may be responsible. In both cases, polyps hinder nasal breathing, impair smell and may increase the risk of asthma. For example, around a third of people with intrinsic asthma suffer from sinusitis and nasal polyps. And 39 per cent of people with aspirin-induced asthma have intrinsic asthma and nasal polyps. So you may want to discuss your options for treating chronic sinusitis and nasal polyps with your doctor.

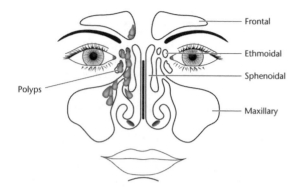

Figure 3.1(a) The sinuses and polyps – front view

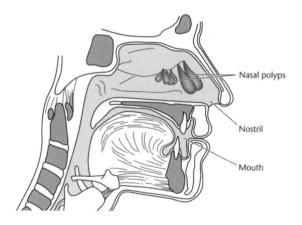

Figure 3.1(b) The sinuses and polyps – side view

Heartburn

Most of us regard a bout of heartburn as the inevitable price for overindulging in spicy or fatty food, alcohol or caffeine, or as yet another consequence of smoking. Indeed, around a third of UK adults have endured the discomfort of heartburn at least once in the last six months. Around a quarter of adults experience heartburn at least monthly and 5 per cent suffer heartburn daily. Furthermore, between 10 and 20 per cent of adults experience GORD, one common cause of heartburn, on at least one day a week. However, people over 65 years of age seem to be especially likely to develop GORD. But don't underestimate this common problem.

Don't dismiss dyspepsia

Dyspepsia can arise from several causes, from overindulgence to potentially fatal cancers. So, if you start experiencing unexplained and persistent heartburn it's worth seeking your GP's advice, especially if you're aged 55 years or older, or experience other symptoms, such as unintentional weight loss, difficulty swallowing, vomiting or signs of anaemia. And GORD occasionally causes potentially serious complications, including:

- strictures (abnormal narrowing) in the food pipe (oesophagus) that cause swallowing difficulties;
- ulcers in the oesophagus (food pipe);
- a condition called Barrett's oesophagus, where damage to the food pipe results in potentially cancerous cells replacing healthy cells in the lower oesophagus.

Barrett's oesophagus is an influential risk factor for a type of cancer called oesophageal adenocarcinoma (OAC). According to Cancer Research UK, between 0.5 and 2 per cent of adults in Western countries probably have Barrett's oesophagus. About 0.5 to 1 per cent of these develop OAC each year. While the absolute risk may be low, patients with Barrett's oesophagus remain 30 to 125 times more likely to develop OAC than the general population.

GORD occurs when the stomach's contents enter the oesophagus. Normally, a valve (sphincter) at the junction of the stomach and oesophagus prevents this 'reflux'. However, certain meals, changes in posture (especially lying down), certain medications (including some drugs used to treat asthma – see page 43) and stress may weaken the sphincter, allowing reflux. As almost everyone suffers indigestion occasionally, gastroenterologists usually diagnose GORD only if patients suffer heartburn on at least one day each week.

Heartburn, GORD's main manifestation, arises as the stomach's contents burn the oesophagus. However, other symptoms include:

- regurgitation of food or acid;
- waterbrash – regurgitation of watery sour or tasteless acid;
- a sudden gush of saliva;
- chest pain;

- cough;
- hoarseness or sore throat;
- bloating, belching, nausea.

Apart from causing some symptoms reminiscent of asthma (such as cough), people with GORD may regurgitate small amounts of stomach acid into their mouths, from where it can seep into their tracheas and lungs. Reflux is especially likely when you lie flat – gravity no longer helps prevent regurgitation. So GORD patients with asthma are especially likely to experience night-time wheezing, breathlessness and cough, and to produce phlegm in the morning. Indeed, Calhoun noted that 9 per cent of GORD patients had asthma, more than twice the number in subjects without GORD (4 per cent). GORD may also exacerbate the variation in lung function and the airway obstruction in people with asthma.

Certain people find that treating GORD relieves some symptoms of their asthma (particularly a bothersome cough). A review of trials by Gibson and colleagues that examined the link between asthma and GORD reported that omeprazole (a drug that reduces acid production by the stomach) improved FEV_1 (a measure of lung function – see Chapter 5) by 20 per cent in four of 14 people with asthma. Overall, the average improvement was 10 per cent. Studies using other anti-reflux drugs failed to find any improvement in lung function. However, asthma symptoms – such as limitation of activity, shortness of breath and wheezing – can improve without objective improvements in lung function. So it's certainly worth treating dyspepsia.

You can buy omeprazole and some other GORD treatments over the counter from pharmacists. Doctors can prescribe higher doses of these drugs and offer a wider choice of treatments for GORD. So, if you feel that GORD is making your symptoms worse, talk to your pharmacist or doctor. (But always let them know you have asthma.) You can also make some lifestyle changes that may alleviate GORD:

- Obesity, smoking, alcohol, coffee and chocolate may transiently relax the sphincter. Fatty foods may slow the rate at which the stomach empties. Both of these changes can contribute to GORD. That's yet another good reason to lose weight, quit smoking and eat a healthy diet.
- As lying flat often makes matters worse, some people find that raising the head of the bed alleviates GORD. (You could try propping the head of your bed up on bricks.)
- You should also avoid eating close to your bedtime. Food stimulates your stomach to produce acid.

Asthma drugs and GORD

Certain treatments for asthma can exacerbate GORD. For example, beta-agonists, anticholinergics and theophylline alleviate asthma symptoms by relaxing the ring of muscle surrounding the airways. But the same mechanism means that they can also relax the sphincter in the lower oesophagus, allowing reflux and triggering GORD. If lifestyle measures don't help, talk to your GP.

Steroid tablets can cause indigestion and ulcers. Some ulcers burn through the wall of the gut or stomach, causing bleeding or even allowing the contents of the gastrointestinal tract to enter the abdomen. However, relatively few people develop these serious side effects. Conn and Poynard reported that three people in 1,000 (0.3 per cent) developed a peptic ulcer (one that hasn't burnt all the way through the wall) while taking an inactive placebo. Oral corticosteroids increased the proportion to 0.4 per cent. In other words, one extra person taking oral steroids developed peptic ulcers for every 1,000 treated. So, if you develop heartburn while taking oral steroids, see your doctor or asthma nurse.

Indoor and outdoor pollution

The World Health Organization (WHO) estimates that outdoor and indoor pollution causes approximately two million premature deaths worldwide per year. Pollution from traffic and factories probably doesn't cause asthma. However, pollution can trigger asthma exacerbations, partly by enhancing the effect of allergens.

While most people think of pollution as the toxic cocktail belching from cars, lorries and factories, we're also exposed to pollution inside our homes, such as smoke from tobacco and (if you use them) coal or wood for heating and cooking. Indoor pollution can also contribute to poor asthma control. After all, we spend at least 75 per cent of our time indoors.

Smoke

Tobacco smoke is probably the most important indoor pollutant for people with asthma. You don't even need to be a tobacco addict to suffer. Passive smoking accounts for around one in every 100 deaths worldwide, according to *The Lancet*. Indeed, passive smoking in the home kills around 11,000 people every year in the UK alone, through lung cancer, stroke and heart disease. Passive smoking can also trigger bronchoconstriction and exacerbate asthma. Second-hand smoke caused 36,900 deaths worldwide from asthma during 2004, *The Lancet* reported. Active smoking, of course, poses an even greater hazard:

- People with asthma who smoke regularly tend to endure more severe symptoms, have a worse quality of life, make more trips to A&E departments and are more likely to need hospitalization than asthmatics who do not smoke.
- Smoking accelerates the decline in lung function compared with people with asthma who do not smoke. Indeed, FEV_1 (a measure of lung function – see Chapter 5) can decline more rapidly in non-allergic cigarette smokers than among people with allergic asthma. On the other hand, quitting smoking can reduce the age-related decline in FEV_1 to that typical among lifelong non-smokers.
- Smokers are more susceptible than non-smokers to infections with rhinoviruses – a group of around 100 viruses that frequently cause common colds – partly because chemicals in tobacco seem to suppress the immune system. So the virus replicates more readily in smoke-damaged than in healthy cells in the lungs. The smoke-damaged cells are more likely to die during the infection.
- Smoking tobacco or marijuana can cause symptoms similar to asthma, which can complicate diagnosis.

We'll look at some ways to quit smoking in Chapter 7.

Smoking in pregnancy

Mums-to-be who smoke are more likely than those who don't to experience problems during pregnancy, including miscarriage, premature birth, stillbirth, low birth weight babies and sudden infant death syndrome. Indeed, smoking during pregnancy increases infant mortality by around 40 per cent. Furthermore, children exposed to tobacco smoke while in the womb are more likely to experience serious respiratory infections (e.g. bronchitis and pneumonia), *Otitis media* (glue ear) and other ear, nose and throat ailments, psychological and behaviour problems and asthma as they grow up.

So the sooner you quit smoking, the better for you and your baby. The intense medical and social pressure against tobacco use in pregnancy makes some women reluctant to admit they smoke. However, for the sake of your baby and yourself, you need help. Your midwife or doctor should be able to offer you advice and support to quit. You could also call the NHS Pregnancy Smoking Helpline number: 0800 169 9 169.

Outdoor pollution

During the London smog in the winter of 1952, a mixture of fog, smoke and chemical fumes hung so thickly in the air that people could barely see a few yards in front of their faces. The smog claimed at least 3,000 to 4,000 lives in addition to those normally expected at that time of the year. Depending on how many people died because of the smog in the early months of 1953, the pollution could have killed as many as 12,000 people, Bell and colleagues estimate. The public outcry led to the 1956 Clean Air Act.

Air quality in the UK has improved over the last 60 years – at the same time as the number of people with asthma has risen. So, rather than *causing* asthma, air pollution tends to exacerbating existing respiratory diseases. For example, people living in towns and cities seem to be more likely to develop asthma due to pollen than those in the country. In part, townies are at increased risk because pollution exacerbates pollen's ability to trigger an immune reaction.

Pollution is a complex cocktail of chemicals, which complicates analysis of the biological effects. Nevertheless, we know that many pollutants, alone or in combination, potentially exacerbate asthma. For example:

- Nitrogen dioxide – a gas produced by cars, gas cookers or heating and power stations – irritates the lining of the lungs and nose.
- Sulphur dioxide – produced by power stations, diesel engines and coal fires – caused most of the respiratory problems during the 1952 smog. Sulphur dioxide can trigger bronchoconstriction.
- Ozone forms when sunlight reacts with nitrogen dioxide and some other pollutants. High ozone levels can cause breathing problems, trigger asthma and reduce lung function.

Many weather forecasts now predict the level of air pollution. When air pollution is high, people with asthma could experience discomfort or symptoms, so they should spend less time outdoors. It's also a good idea to avoid exercising in front of an open window. Pollution levels are also much higher in other parts of the world than in the UK; it might be worth checking the air quality of any city you plan to visit before you decide whether to book your tickets.

Indoor pollution

With cars and lorries belching out toxic fumes, it's easy to forget the risks posed by indoor air pollution. But most of us spend far more time indoors than outside, so our cumulative exposure to indoor pollution is greater. Again, several sources of indoor pollution can exacerbate asthma:

- Levels of nitrogen dioxide produced by gas cookers and kerosene heaters inside the house can be higher than those produced outside by cars and power stations.
- Open fires and paraffin stoves can produce high levels of sulphur dioxide and particulate pollutants.
- Particulate matter released during cooking and by aerosols can reduce lung function and increase the risk of heart and lung diseases. Stir-frying, for example, creates a high concentration of particulate matter, including superheated oil particles.
- Numerous sources – including some DIY products, cleaning products, air fresheners, paints and electrical goods – release natural and synthetic volatile organic compounds (such as formaldehyde). These may irritate the respiratory tract and possibly exacerbate asthma. Volatile organic compounds also react with ozone (produced indoors by some printers). The reaction generates other compounds that potentially undermine lung function.

Weather

On 6 and 7 July 1983, doctors in Birmingham treated 26 emergency cases of asthma over 36 hours, compared to the expected two or three a day. On 24 June 1994, A&E departments across London and southwest England managed 640 people with asthma and other respiratory diseases over 30 hours, almost ten times the expected number. On both occasions, D'Amato and colleagues comment, heavy thunderstorms swept the areas.

Since then, doctors as far away as Italy and Australia have reported a surge in the number of asthma cases during thunderstorms. D'Amato and colleagues suggest that thunderstorms concentrate pollen at ground level. The atmospheric conditions then cause the pollen to burst, producing aerosols of highly allergenic particles that – because of their small size – penetrate deep into the lower airways. In sensitive people, the high concentration of allergen triggers asthma. Indeed, people with allergic rhinitis caused by pollen ('hay fever') who do not normally experience respiratory symptoms can suffer full-blown asthma attacks during some thunderstorms. (Remember that, in effect, the respiratory tract is a single organ running from the nose to the alveoli.)

Thunderstorm-asthma seems to be rare. But the weather can affect the risk of suffering asthma and other allergies in other ways.

- We've already seen that cold air commonly triggers asthma.
- Ozone levels rise on sunny days, and this, as we've seen, can trigger asthma.
- Certain weather patterns increase pollen release. Most flowers

release pollen in the early morning, often triggered by changes in humidity. On the other hand, rain can remove pollen from the air.

So, if you think a particular weather pattern exacerbates your symptoms, try to limit your exposure at these times.

Finally, climate change may alter the long-term profile of allergens. For instance, American researchers have noted a rise in levels of ragweed pollen, fungal spores and poison ivy in recent years, which they attribute to rising levels of carbon dioxide in the atmosphere. The rise in carbon dioxide levels feeds the plant, which may prompt increased pollen production. The increased plant activity also offers fungi living on the leaves the opportunity to reproduce more rapidly and increase spore production.

Inside the house, climate change can increase humidity, which may encourage the proliferation of dust mite and mould. High temperature and humidity also speeds the decomposition of food, which is a feast for certain insects, some of which can trigger asthma in sensitive people. Cockroaches, for example, are a particularly common asthma trigger in the USA and some parts of Europe. (So avoid piles of papers and keep food in airtight containers to help control cockroaches.)

Poor adherence

The most effective drug is useless unless you take it correctly. That sounds obvious. Yet Clatworthy and colleagues found that, in the UK, a third of adults with asthma admitted poor adherence with their treatment. (The terms 'poor compliance' or 'poor concordance' also describe patients who don't take their medicines as agreed with their doctor or nurse.) In another study, Bozek and Jarzab found that only between 9 and 21 per cent of patients aged 65 to 102 years with chronic asthma adhered well to their therapy.

There are a variety of reasons people with asthma may not adhere to medicines that could save their life. Some may deny that they are ill, disbelieve the diagnosis, have low expectations of treatment, suffer from psychiatric problems (Chapter 7) or fail to appreciate the risks associated with poor compliance. Others may comply poorly because they are worried about side effects or because treatment disrupts their lifestyle unacceptably. If this sounds like you, have an open and honest discussion about your concerns with your GP or asthma nurse.

Some people also take excessive amounts of their drugs – perhaps overdosing on steroid or bronchodilator – usually through fear that they'll suffer a serious attack. Again, a full and frank discussion with your doctor or nurse should help you place the risks in perspective. In such cases, a self-management plan will often help to put you back in control and allow you to increase the dose of medication when your symptoms or peak flow worsen.

Often, however, poor adherence is unintentional. People may misunderstand treatment instructions, become confused over their medicines – especially if they suffer from other diseases and need to take several drugs – or simply forget. In these cases, adherence aids (such as a box that allows you to organize your tablets day by day) could help, as could simplifying your treatment and asking your doctor to check that you really need all the drugs. You could try keeping your steroid by your bedside if you need to take your anti-inflammatory twice a day. (Obviously, keep all medicines out of the reach of children.) The more drugs you need, the more the chance of poor compliance rises and these aids can help you remember to take your treatment on time.

People with physical disabilities may experience difficulties opening packaging or swallowing medication. Pharmacists may be able to suggest alternative packaging or dosing forms that overcome these limitations, such as avoiding 'child-resistant' pill bottles or using liquid formulations. If you can't use the inhaler correctly, changing the inhaler or using an aid may help.

Finally, other family members and caregivers should understand the cause of and triggers for asthma, as well as the need for effective treatment, especially, for example, if the person is elderly or tends to forget his or her medication. Unintentional poor adherence may become increasingly common with advancing age or in those suffering diseases, such as dementia, that compromise their mental abilities. In such cases, involving family members and other caregivers promotes adherence.

Pregnancy and asthma

The *British Guideline for Asthma Management* (which we'll discuss further in Chapter 6; see Useful addresses) notes that poorly controlled asthma increases the risk of numerous complications for the baby and the mother, including:

- hyperemesis (sickness, especially in the morning);
- pre-eclampsia (dangerously raised blood pressure – hypertension – during pregnancy);
- vaginal haemorrhage;
- complications during labour;
- foetal growth restriction (poor growth of the developing baby) – in

one study, suffering asthma symptoms daily increased the risk of poor foetal growth by 125 per cent;

- low birth weight – one study found that suffering asthma exacerbations during pregnancy increased the risk of low birth weight by 154 per cent;
- premature birth;
- increased risk of death immediately before and just after birth (the perinatal period);
- neonatal hypoxia (lack of oxygen to the baby), which can cause cerebral palsy, blindness and epilepsy as well as impairing mental and psychomotor development.

This is a worrying list. But it's important to remember that most women with asthma have normal pregnancies and, provided their symptoms are well controlled, the risk of complications is small, the *British Guideline on Asthma Management* notes. Indeed, asthma often improves during pregnancy.

Obviously, the mother's body undergoes numerous, often profound, changes during pregnancy, some of which could worsen or improve asthma. One study found that asthma worsened during pregnancy in 35 per cent of women. Another study found that asthma improved and deteriorated in 23 and 30 per cent respectively. So, broadly, asthma improves in one-third of women during pregnancy; a third of mums-to-be finds that their asthma symptoms worsen; and symptoms don't change in the final third of expectant mothers.

Severe asthma is more likely to worsen during pregnancy than mild asthma. Nevertheless, symptoms may improve during pregnancy in some women with serious symptoms and deteriorate in some with mild asthma. Asthma is also most likely to worsen during the second and third trimesters, with the risk reaching a peak during the sixth month. The risk of suffering an exacerbation appears to be lowest during the last month of pregnancy. But changes can emerge almost any time during the nine months.

Short-acting bronchodilators (relievers) control most exacerbations during pregnancy. Nevertheless, 11 to 18 per cent of expectant mothers with asthma will suffer at least one exacerbation during their pregnancy that needs treatment in an A&E department. Of these, 62 per cent will require hospitalization. This unpredictability and the risks to you and your baby mean that it is especially important to monitor your peak flow and symptoms during pregnancy.

Breast-feeding and asthma

Breast-feeding may lower a child's risk of suffering from asthma, partly by reducing exposure to food allergens in early infancy. Indeed, breast-feeding seems to reduce the risk that infants will develop asthma, regardless of whether one or both parents suffered from allergies. Nevertheless, breast-feeding's protective effect is most marked in high-risk infants (for example, because their parents suffered from severe allergies). However, mothers need to breast-feed the baby for at least four months to gain the maximum protection.

Menstrual cycles and asthma

Many women find that their asthma symptoms worsen just before their period. Estimates vary from study to study, depending partly on the definitions used. Some researchers suggest that up to 40 per cent of women experience premenopausal asthma. Murphy and Gibson found that 57 per cent of women showed premenstrual increases in symptoms and asthma medication use. However, only 25 per cent experienced premenstrual exacerbations in each of the cycles studied. Dratva and co-researchers found that women were 2.3 times more likely to show increased bronchial hyper-reactivity in the three days before and the same time after the first day of menstruation, compared to other times in their cycle. So premenstrual asthma is certainly common.

As you might expect, changes in hormone levels underlie these premenopausal exacerbations, which do not seem to depend on whether or not the woman suffers from allergic or intrinsic asthma, and there is no clear link with symptom severity. Levels of the sex hormones oestrogen and progesterone during the menstrual cycle seem to increase bronchial reactivity, partly by altering the activity of beta$_2$-receptors (responsible for controlling airway calibre) and possibly by increasing levels of leukotrienes, an inflammatory mediator (we'll hear more about both of these in Chapter 6). Oestrogen may also reduce the body's production of natural anti-inflammatory chemicals.

Asthmatic worsening before the period appears to be associated with other aspects of the premenstrual syndrome. Pereira-Vega and colleagues found that 45 per cent of women reported a premenstrual worsening of respiratory symptoms, peak flow or both. These women were also more likely to report premenstrual dysphoria (feelings such as anxiety, depression, fatigue, irritability and mood swings) and sensations of swelling or tension in their abdomen, breasts and elsewhere. This supports the idea that hormonal changes cause premenstrual exacerbations.

Inhaled steroids may be less effective against perimenstrual asthma worsenings (those around the period) than in other exacerbations. As rising leukotriene levels may contribute to premenstrual asthma, Dean argues that adding a drug that specifically blocks these mediators – a leukotriene receptor antagonist (see Chapter 6) – might be a better treatment choice than increasing the steroid dose. Some (but not all) studies suggest that oral contraceptives lessen the increase in bronchial hyper-reactivity around the time of your period and protect against premenstrual asthma. You could try keeping a diary recording your periods and peak flow as well as asthmatic and perimenstrual symptoms. If this reveals a worsening around the time of your period, discuss your treatment choices with your doctor or asthma nurse.

Asthma and the menopause

Some women develop asthma for the first time after their menopause, especially if they are overweight. And the risk of developing asthma in postmenopausal women rises the more pounds they pile on. Furthermore, some forms of hormone replacement therapy (HRT) may trigger asthma. (This isn't surprising – we've already seen that hormonal changes probably underlie menstrual asthma.) For example, Romieu and colleagues found that using HRT containing oestrogen alone or oestrogen plus progestin (a synthetic progestogen) doubled the risk of developing asthma. However, another study found that only those who used HRT containing oestrogen alone were at increased risk (a 54 per cent rise), particularly if they had never smoked (80 per cent rise) or suffered allergic disease before asthma's onset (86 per cent increase).

The differences between the studies suggest that HRT's effects on asthma vary in different subgroups of women. If you feel that you need HRT, for example to treat hot flushes, night sweats, vaginal symptoms and cystitis, you may want to discuss the potential impact on your asthma with your GP. In some cases, there may be alternative ways to manage your symptoms.

4

Occupational asthma

Doctors first linked certain occupations with respiratory problems during the eighteenth century. Today, we know that at least 350 agents used in the workplace may trigger occupational asthma. For example, Henneberger and colleagues remark that high levels of biological dust increase the likelihood of an asthma exacerbation almost four-fold. Low levels of biological dust and high levels of mineral dust almost double the risk.

As occupational asthma often shows a clear pattern of onset and the symptoms frequently improve when exposure to the trigger ceases (such as during holidays), many cases are potentially preventable. Certain countries – including the UK and some parts of the USA – monitor occupational lung diseases, including asthma. Nevertheless, estimates of the number of people affected by work-related asthma vary widely. Scientists who study patterns of diseases (epidemiologists) suggest that work-related factors probably cause between a tenth and a quarter of asthma cases among adults. However, Henneberger and colleagues point out that doctors may have diagnosed only a third of occupational asthma cases. And people who suffer respiratory symptoms may voluntarily change job, leading epidemiologists to further underestimate the true risk.

Parental occupation and childhood asthma

Certain parental occupations seem to increase the likelihood that their children will wheeze or suffer asthma. Parents can transport potential hazards – including pesticides, organic solvents and allergens (such as wheat, latex and dander from laboratory animals) from work to home. This potentially exposes children and other household members to the trigger.

The three routes to occupational asthma

Broadly, occupational factors can trigger asthma in three ways. First, as we saw in Chapter 1, certain allergens sensitize the immune system and prompt production of large amounts of specific IgE. This takes time. So asthma symptoms arising from sensitization to occupational allergens tend to emerge several months or even years after exposure starts.

Once the worker's immune system generates specific IgE, exposure to very low levels of the occupational trigger can provoke symptoms.

Second, chemicals that irritate the lining of the lung, damage the bronchial wall or increase the number of inflammatory cells can trigger asthma. Indeed, a single exposure to high levels of some airway irritants can cause this 'non-allergic' occupational asthma. In one case, Kern reports, 21 per cent of hospital workers exposed to high levels of acetic acid following a spill developed irritant-induced asthma. This compared with 3 per cent of those with medium levels of exposure to acetic acid and none of those exposed to low levels. Similarly, exposure to high levels of gas and fumes increases the risk of suffering asthma two and a half times. One study found that a fire, mixing cleaning agents and a chemical spill each trebled asthma risk.

In contrast to the allergic form, this form of asthma develops minutes or hours after a usually recognizable incident (such as a fire or chemical spill) during which the worker was exposed to high levels of a respiratory irritant. In many cases, the person had not previously suffered respiratory disease. Indeed, workers often report many years of exposure to low levels of the agent without suffering symptoms. In other cases, frequent lower-intensity exposures to certain chemicals may induce asthma, although further studies need to determine how many cases arise from this mechanism.

Finally, various non-specific factors – such as dust, cold air and physical exercise – at work can provoke pre-existing asthma or undermine lung function. Images of a cloud of dust sweeping through Manhattan's streets following the terrorist attacks on the World Trade Center on September 11, 2001, remain unforgettable. Not surprisingly, lung function declined markedly in rescue workers exposed to the dust. Aldrich and colleagues found that in the year after the attack, mean FEV_1 (see Chapter 5) fell by 439 ml and 267 ml in fire fighters and emergency medical service workers respectively who had never smoked. Lung function improved little during the next six years. After six years, 13 per cent of fire fighters and 22 per cent of emergency medical service workers showed FEV_1 below the lower limit of the normal range. This extreme example illustrates that chemically and biologically 'inert' dust can still cause considerable lung damage.

Cigarette smoking further increases the risk of sensitization or asthma symptoms in several workforces, while some chemicals may directly contract bronchial smooth muscle. Finally, people with manual jobs may find that exercise triggers symptoms. In these cases, the treatments for exercise-induced asthma (Chapter 2) may help.

Common causes of occupational asthma

Almost every occupation is at risk of exposure to factors that trigger or exacerbate asthma, even that of office worker – some printers produce ozone, for example. Nevertheless, people working in certain occupations are at especially high risk of developing work-related asthma, as the following examples illustrate.

Bakers and flourmill workers

The Italian physician Bernardino Ramazzini first linked asthma with working in a bakery in his book *De Morbis Artificum Diatriba* [Diseases of Workers] published in 1713. Doctors now know that numerous factors in a bakery can cause sensitization and, in some cases, asthma; these include: wheat, rye, barley, oat and other flours; α-amylase (an enzyme that helps yeast work); and contaminants such as mites and fungi. Indeed, in dusty areas of bakeries and flourmills, up to 20 per cent of airborne allergen particles are small enough to deposit in bronchioles and alveoli.

The variety of allergens responsible for occupational asthma among bakers continues to expand. Most people think of lupins as ornamental flowers. But lupins belong to the legume family of plants, alongside peanuts, peas, chickpeas and lentils. Indeed, lupin beans (*lupini*) are a traditional dish in some Mediterranean countries and were cultivated in the Roman Empire. Today, lupin products – such as flour – are increasingly used to manufacture bread, pasta and pastries and to thicken soup.

Campbell and Yates point out that, despite centuries of its use, the first reports of occupational sensitization to lupin emerged only in 2001. Since then, studies have suggested that between 21 and 29 per cent of people who inhale lupin at work become sensitized. Lupin allergies can cause asthma, conjunctivitis (an inflammatory reaction on the outermost surface of the eye and the inside of the eyelid) and rhinitis. As this example illustrates, it's important to remain vigilant for changes in asthma patterns when your company introduces new processes.

Enzymes

Detergent manufacturers, food processors (including bakers), research staff and healthcare professionals use enzymes, which, as they're proteins, can evoke allergic reactions. Workers manufacturing enzymes and detergent products seem to be at the highest risk. But even lower levels can cause respiratory symptoms. Kitchen staff using papain to tenderize meat can become sensitized and develop respiratory disease, for example. Indeed, any protein that can become airborne and is of a size that can deposit in the lower airways could probably induce occupational asthma in some people.

Chemicals

Numerous chemicals can cause or trigger asthma, including complex platinum salts (used in the refining of precious metals, the chemical and pharmaceutical industries) and a group of compounds called diisocyanates. Many of these chemicals are much smaller than protein allergens. However, platinum salts, diisocyanates and some other chemicals seem to bind to, and change the shape of, proteins produced naturally by the body. The immune system produces antibodies against these altered proteins. And some chemicals – such as certain diisocyanates – may contract the muscles around the airways.

Diisocyanates are used to manufacture polyurethane. As polyurethanes are widely used, workers can be exposed to diisocyanates when applying certain paints (such as aircraft and car spray paints) and from some inks and adhesives, for example. There are several diisocyanates, each of which can cause occupational asthma. In Europe, hexamethylene diisocyanate used in spray paints probably accounts for most cases of occupational asthma caused by this group of chemicals. Sensitive workers can react to minute amounts of diisocyanates. For example, workers sensitized to toluene diisocyanate may develop asthma after exposure to concentrations as low as one part in a billion.

Wood dust

Wood dust is another potential cause of occupational asthma. For example, Schlünssen and colleagues found that 1.7 and 3.1 per cent of woodworkers in furniture factories showed IgE to pine and beech respectively. Although the risk was relatively low, the likelihood of being sensitized rose as exposure to wood dust increased.

Similarly, Campo and colleagues found that 54 per cent of carpentry apprentices had work-related respiratory symptoms caused by wood dust, 15 per cent due to diisocyanate and 9 per cent to both. Those who suffered from rhinitis were roughly twice as likely to develop respiratory symptoms due to wood dust exposure compared to those without rhinitis. In asthmatic apprentices, the risk of respiratory symptoms due to wood dust was almost three times higher. In this study, 9 per cent of participants showed specific IgE to wood.

Workers handling animals

As we saw in Chapter 2, dander and other allergens from domestic pets are common causes of allergic asthma. Allergens in urine, pelt, hair and blood also contribute to occupational asthma among people working with animals. Indeed, 28 per cent of airborne allergens liberated from rat urine in animal laboratories are tiny enough to deposit in the small airways. Larger particles may deposit in the nose, which can provoke occupational rhinitis.

Overall, around 15 per cent of workers become sensitized and about 2 per cent develop asthma during their first year of working with animals. Another way to look at the risk calculates the number of cases per person-month: so, 12 people working for one month and one person working for 12 months both represent 12 person-months. Positive skin tests (see Chapter 5) to rat urine develop at a rate of approximately 2.5 new cases per 1,000 person-months.

Latex allergies

Latex is the milky sap from the rubber tree. Manufacturers process latex to create, among many other products, adhesives, foam, carpet backings, medical gloves, catheters, condoms and balloons. Unfortunately, natural latex contains numerous allergens that sensitive people may inhale or absorb through their mucosa – such as people who need indwelling urinary catheters – and possibly skin. People who need to change latex gloves regularly (such as healthcare workers) seem to be at higher risk of developing sensitivity to latex. Furthermore, people sensitive to natural rubber latex may cross-react to several foods and plants, including avocados, bananas and the weeping fig (*Ficus benjamina*).

Colophony

Colophony, a resin produced by pine trees, is used as a solder flux and, less commonly, as a coolant, in bitumen and in poultry processing. Soldering releases a fume of acids and other chemicals that can, when inhaled, trigger asthma in some patients. In one study, around a fifth of patients working in areas of a factory with high levels of colophony fumes developed work-related respiratory symptoms. This compared to between 4 and 16 per cent in other parts of the factory. However, exactly how colophony triggers asthma isn't clear.

Horticulture

Not surprisingly, given its importance as an allergen in the general population, pollen can trigger asthma among people working in horticulture. Patiwael and colleagues, for example, found that, over eight years, 9 per cent of people working growing bell (sweet) peppers in greenhouses produced IgE to the pollen. Furthermore, 19 per cent showed work-related rhinitis. In this study, atopy (a genetic tendency to develop allergies, see Chapter 1) and smoking increased the risk of developing occupational rhinitis by approximately six and four times respectively. Moreover, 8 per cent of workers in horticulture showed work-related asthma symptoms, with atopy and smoking increasing the risk by five and almost twelve times respectively.

Pollen isn't the only potential occupational trigger in horticulture. For example, spider mites – a pest affecting various crops grown in greenhouses and fruit orchards – can trigger allergy and asthma in greenhouse workers, farmers and children living in rural areas. Because of concerns about the safety of pesticides among consumers, some growers have started using predatory mites to hunt down the pests. However, anti-pest mites can prove allergenic. Kronqvist and colleagues found that 36 per cent of people working in greenhouses growing cucumbers and tomatoes were sensitized to at least one predatory or pest mite species. Of these, 35 per cent had asthma and 47 per cent suffered from rhinitis and conjunctivitis.

Diagnosing occupational asthma

It's vital to get the diagnosis right: people suffering from occupational asthma usually need to change their job or may even face unemployment. On average, according to Ayres and co-authors, changing jobs because of occupational asthma typically reduces income by between 22 and 50 per cent. Indeed, between 20 and 80 per cent of those who change job suffer some loss of income.

Unfortunately, you can't rely on your inhalers to stay at work. Standard asthma treatments may not work optimally if the allergen exposure continues. Protective equipment – such as air-fed helmet respirators – may improve or abolish symptoms in some employees. However, these can be uncomfortable and cumbersome.

So how can you tell whether you encounter the trigger for your asthma at home, at work or at play? If you suffer asthma symptoms (e.g. cough and chest tightness) at work but these are absent or less severe after work, at weekends or while on holiday, you may suffer from occupational or work-exacerbated asthma.

However, this pattern isn't infallible. The late-phase reaction (Chapter 1) means that asthmatic symptoms can occur during the evening or night following exposure. Furthermore, on repeated exposure, people with oc-cupational asthma take longer to recover. So symptoms may not improve over the weekend, but abate only after you've been on holiday for several days. To complicate matters further, non-specific triggers – including cold air, tobacco smoke, exhaust fumes and the vapours of paint or perfumes – can cause symptoms at home, even if the cause is work-based.

If the doctor suspects that you suffer from work-related asthma, you'll probably be asked to measure your lung function at home and at work. And it's a good idea to keep a diary of your known exposures at work. You may also undergo a challenge test or other investigations (such as a skin prick test) to see if you have become sensitized (see Chapter 5).

Tests to detect specific IgE antibodies can support the diagnosis. But used alone the tests are rarely sufficient to diagnose asthma. Antibodies indicate only that the person is 'sensitized' and not that the particular trigger causes your symptoms. Many more people are sensitized than develop asthma or other allergic symptoms. Nevertheless, doctors may suggest a diagnosis of occupational asthma based on very high antibody levels (called titres) in people with a characteristic pattern of symptoms. The next chapter considers these tests.

Most occupational asthma improves once exposure to the allergen ends. But while many recover completely, some find that their asthmatic symptoms and airway hyper-reactivity do not resolve. And some people who develop work-related asthma endure persistent symptoms despite avoiding the occupational allergen.

One group of researchers, led by Rachiotis, examined 39 studies investigating outcomes in occupational asthma. A third of people recovered completely from their asthma over an average of 31 months. However, in individual studies recovery rates varied from zero to 100 per cent. Furthermore, 73 per cent of patients showed non-specific bronchial hyper-responsiveness. Workers with the longest durations of employment or symptomatic exposure were the least likely to recover, possibly reflecting the impact of airway remodelling.

Not surprisingly, doctors and employers have looked for ways to reduce the risk of occupational asthma. The 30 to 40 per cent of the population who are atopic (see Chapter 1) are especially likely to develop occupational asthma from, among others triggers, allergens in a bakery, animals, detergent enzymes, certain dyes and some seafoods. However, most atopic subjects will develop neither sensitization nor asthma symptoms. So, for example, in order to prevent one asthma case a laboratory would need to exclude seven atopic employees who could handle the animals. The difficulty predicting who is at risk means asthma remains an occupational hazard for millions of workers.

5

Diagnosing asthma in adults

Asthmatics fear the hallmark breathlessness, chest pain and cough. Yet symptoms alone are not always a reliable means of diagnosing and monitoring asthma. For instance, breathlessness on exercise may be unreliable as a guide to severity if adults walk more slowly as breathing becomes more difficult. Furthermore, asthma symptoms correlate poorly with objective measurements of lung function and the severity of the underlying inflammation. Indeed, some people with severe asthma report fewer and less intense symptoms than people with milder asthma.

Moreover, at any given severity, older people typically feel that their symptoms are more severe than younger people. Ekici and collaborators found that older people with asthma (average age 67 years) show similar lung function to younger people (average age 42 years). However, most older people with asthma reported feeling more breathless when they exercised. Older people also tend to feel that a similar exacerbation is more severe compared to the perception of younger patients. On the other hand, older people are typically less able to perceive bronchoconstriction following exposure to chemicals than younger asthmatics. So older people may not appreciate the seriousness of the attack.

Other factors complicate the relationship between symptoms and asthma severity. For example, older people may regard limitations to their activity as inevitable (because of their asthma, age or both) and not necessarily a marker of poor control. For instance, a review in *The Lancet* reports that up to a third of older people report feeling breathless – but around 70 per cent of these regard breathlessness as a normal part of ageing, so they don't report symptoms that they regard as 'normal' to their GP or asthma nurse. This leads to under-treatment, and therefore to more severe symptoms.

Finally, asthma's symptoms overlap with those of other diseases common in older people, which complicates diagnosis and treatment. For example, the *Lancet* review reports that 14 per cent of people over the age of 75 years wheezed. COPD, heart failure, acute bronchitis, bronchiectasis (abnormal widening of the airways), cancer and pulmonary embolism (caused when a clot blocks a blood vessel supplying the lung) can cause wheeze. Partly because of these problems, doctors have not diagnosed asthma in about half of the elderly people who suffer from the condition. As a consequence, the patients endure unnecessary symptoms.

Lung function tests

Because of the weak association between severity and symptoms, doctors use 'lung function tests' to diagnose asthma, monitor response to treatment and offer an early warning of an impending attack. Several factors influence lung function, including the following:

- Lung capacity is about a fifth to a quarter lower in women compared with men, even if they're the same height and weight.
- Normally, lung function increases until early adolescence and then remains stable until the patient's mid-30s. Lung function then declines, partly because lungs become less elastic as we get older.
- People who developed asthma for the first time aged over 60 years showed a more rapid decline in FEV_1 – see page 62 – (42 ml a year) than those without asthma (2 ml a year) or those who already had asthma (15 ml a year).

To allow for such factors, doctors usually express the results of lung function tests as a percentage of those predicted for other people of the same age, sex and height based on measurements in thousands of healthy people. Doctors generally regard normal lung function as being within 85 per cent of the predicted average value.

Peak flow

Peak flow measures the maximum rate at which air moves when you exhale. This indirectly indicates the airway's diameter when you breathe out. Despite the fact that you exhale for only a second or two, doctors measure peak flow in litres per minute.

Peak flow measurements can offer valuable insights into your asthma. For instance, an improvement of 60 litres a minute (l/min) or at least 20 per cent after taking a short-acting bronchodilator strongly suggests asthma. Furthermore, when diagnosing asthma your doctor or nurse may ask you to measure your peak flow in the morning and evening (sometimes more frequently) for, usually, a couple of weeks. Asthma patients tend to show a greater variation in their measurements over the course of a day (called the diurnal or circadian variation) than healthy people and those with some other diseases (Figure 5.1). In asthma, the diurnal variation is more than 20 per cent and appears to be especially marked in people with intrinsic, compared to allergic, asthma.

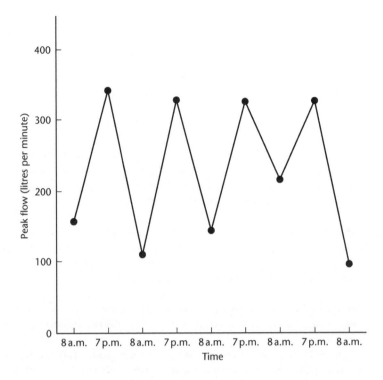

Figure 5.1 Example of a 'saw-tooth' pattern in severe asthma

Keeping a peak flow record

If you keep a peak flow record, either to aid diagnosis or to monitor your disease, it is worth noting symptoms and any triggers (such as exercise or factors at work). This may help you identify a cause. If your symptoms get worse when vacuuming or making beds, you could be allergic to house dust mites or dander, for example. Symptoms that improve when you are away from home for a week or more, then relapse when you return, may suggest you're reacting to an allergen in the house. If the doctor suspects occupational asthma, you may take peak flow measurements at and away from work – such as every two hours over four weeks. However, the duration depends on your particular circumstances, such as how long your symptoms take to improve when you are away from work. It's important to note the hours you're at work, to allow for shift patterns, for example.

In general, asthma symptoms do not emerge until peak flow declines by 25 per cent or more from your personal best. So, regularly measuring peak flow can offer an early warning of an impending exacerbation and helps ensure your asthma is well controlled. In general, if peak flow is commonly a third or more below your best, your asthma may be poorly controlled. For example, if your predicted peak flow is 500 l/min:

- a value of 400 l/min means that your asthma may still be well controlled;
- if peak flow drops to 300 l/min you may need to change your treatment (usually by increasing the dose of your inhaled steroid or taking a short course of oral steroid) as part of a self-management plan (Chapter 6) to restore good control.

Likewise, an increase in the normal circadian variation – the difference between the peak and the trough – may indicate poor control, increased severity or both. Nevertheless, peak flow charts may not always accurately reflect asthma's severity. For example:

- Abdominal fat can hinder the diaphragm's descent and, as a result, peak flow declines. So, carrying excessive weight can undermine the chart's accuracy.
- Some healthy people from non-white ethnic groups have different normal peak flow rates from those of Caucasians. Current charts may not account fully for such ethnic differences.
- Factors other than asthma, including tobacco smoke and some other irritants, can influence peak flow.
- Several diseases other than asthma can increase diurnal variation.

Spirometry

Spirometry measures the volume of air expelled in one breath over time, when you breathe out as hard as you can after breathing in as deeply as possible. The forced vital capacity (FVC) is the total volume of air expelled forcefully until no more air can be breathed out. In healthy people, FVC is around 60 per cent of the lungs' total capacity. The remainder represents the residual volume – the amount of air in the airways after a breath (see Figure 5.2).

As you breathe out, the volume of air exhaled initially increases rapidly and then levels off. In general, healthy people take around four seconds to expel a full breath, and usually expel at least 75 per cent of the breath in the first second. Lung disease can reduce this proportion of the breath exhaled, so spirometry allows doctors to calculate 'forced expiratory volume in one second' (FEV_1).

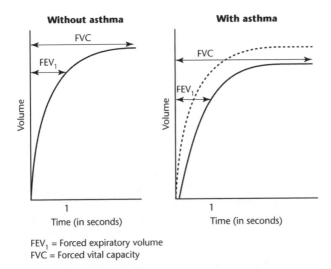

FEV$_1$ = Forced expiratory volume
FVC = Forced vital capacity

Figure 5.2 FEV$_1$ and FVC in people with and without asthma

Doctors calculate the ratio between FEV$_1$ and FVC. In healthy people, the FEV$_1$:FVC ratio is 0.75 (or 75 per cent). People with asthma have narrow airways, so they exhale more slowly and FEV$_1$ declines. FVC also declines, but to a lesser extent than FEV$_1$. For example, an FEV$_1$:FVC ratio of 75 per cent or less of the predicted level is a more sensitive indicator of airway obstruction than peak flow. Indeed, the ratio may decline (indicating obstruction) when FEV$_1$ is normal.

In general, spirometry offers a more accurate measure of lung function than peak flow, depends less on the person's effort and is more reproducible than peak flow. Normal spirometry while you experience symptoms means that it's unlikely you have asthma. On the other hand, spirometry may be normal when you don't have symptoms, so you may have to undergo repeated measurements at the surgery or clinic.

To aid diagnosis, doctors may measure your lung function using the spirometer before and after a dose of short-acting bronchodilator. An improvement in FEV$_1$ of more than 200 to 400 ml (or more than 15 per cent) suggests that the airway's obstruction is reversible, and therefore makes it more likely that you suffer from asthma rather than, for example, COPD (see page 66). However, remodelling means that the lung function of those with chronic severe asthma may not improve to this extent after bronchodilators. In such cases, an improvement after a trial of oral steroids (which potently reduce inflammation) for 14 days often clinches the diagnosis (inflammation is far more important in asthma than COPD).

Challenge tests

As we've noted several times, asthmatic airways constrict when exposed to non-specific triggers such as cold air, dust, aerosol sprays and tobacco smoke. Doctors use this bronchial hyper-reactivity to help diagnose asthma using challenge tests. For example, a chemical called methacholine constricts the airways. The doctor gradually increases the dose of methacholine a person with suspected asthma inhales until FEV_1 declines by 20 per cent. Most asthmatics – around 95 per cent – need a much lower dose of methacholine to constrict their bronchi by 20 per cent than people with healthy lungs. Other challenge tests use histamine, cold air, saline (a salt solution), exercise or adenosine.

However, a challenge test isn't necessarily definitive. Some people with healthy lungs, smokers and many with chronic bronchitis, bronchiectasis or cystic fibrosis show abnormal challenge tests. Moreover, McGrath and Fahy found that 27 per cent of adults diagnosed with asthma by their doctor had a negative methacholine test. Those whose symptoms emerged during adulthood, those with normal FEV_1 and those who did not require oral steroids were especially likely to show negative methacholine tests. Nevertheless, 60 per cent of those with a negative test reported experiencing asthma-like symptoms (cough, dyspnoea – shortness of breath – chest tightness or wheeze) at least once a week. Indeed, 39 per cent said they had visited an A&E department for asthma-like symptoms and 13 per cent had been hospitalized for asthma.

In some cases of suspected occupational asthma, the doctor will ask you to inhale one or more suspected triggers under very carefully controlled conditions. To reduce the risk of a severe attack, the dose is generally lower than the level encountered at work. Nevertheless, challenge tests can be dangerous – there's always the risk that the test will trigger a serious, even life-threatening exacerbation – so specialized centres perform these tests and have equipment and trained staff at hand in case you should develop a severe reaction. During the test, you'll probably also inhale an inert material. You won't know which substance is which until after the test. This allows the doctor to account for any psychological reaction. Not surprisingly, people can be nervous when they undergo challenge tests. And stress can affect your respiration, a point we'll return to in the last chapter.

Immune tests

Because allergies commonly cause asthma, doctors may suggest tests that determine whether your immune system is sensitized to a particular allergen. These tests are more useful to rule out a cause rather than to determine that, for example, grass pollen specifically causes your allergy. If you don't show a positive reaction, the allergen probably isn't responsible. On the other hand, if you test positive that doesn't necessarily mean the allergen is responsible. You may be sensitive – in other words, produce IgE to the allergen – without the immune reaction being sufficiently severe to trigger asthma.

Skin prick tests

Skin prick tests are the longest-established immune investigation. The English scientist Charles Blakely performed the first skin prick test – on himself – in 1869. Blakely wanted to test his idea that pollen caused his hay fever. The test has changed little in more than 140 years.

During a skin prick test, the doctor or nurse uses a fine needle to press a small amount of the suspected allergen into your skin on the inside of your forearm. The needle is held almost parallel to the skin and doesn't go very deep. (I've had this done several times. It doesn't hurt. Really!) A swelling (weal) surrounded by a red flare 15 minutes or so later suggests you're sensitive to that allergen.

The test includes two 'controls': the fluid used to suspend the allergen (called the vehicle) and histamine, to deliberately provoke weal and flare. A reaction to histamine shows the test is working correctly and helps doctors evaluate the results. Some elderly people may show a less marked response to a skin prick test than younger ones, for example. The control ensures that the vehicle doesn't provoke symptoms.

Blood tests

Another type of immune investigation measures levels of IgE circulating in your blood, either the total amount or the concentration specific for a particular allergen. A high level of IgE suggests that an allergy may underlie your asthma. However, a positive test is much more common than symptoms. For example, between 8 and 35 per cent of young adults in Europe show IgE to grass pollen. Nevertheless, the test can rule out allergens and forms one piece in the jigsaw of tests that doctors use to decide whether you're suffering from allergic asthma.

Diagnostic dilemmas

At least half of people aged 65 years and over have three or more co-morbidities, some of which – including COPD, congestive heart failure and vocal cord dysfunction – can mimic asthma's symptoms. Other less common asthma mimics include cystic fibrosis, cancer and bronchiectasis. However, some people have *both* asthma and other diseases that cause similar symptoms, and this considerably complicates diagnosis and treatment. An asthmatic smoker may show signs of COPD, for example. Similarly, heart disease remains the UK's leading killer and many asthmatics suffer a heart attack – simply because both conditions are common. Heart attack (myocardial infarction) survivors are at risk of heart failure, one symptom of which is 'cardiac asthma'. So you may undergo tests to examine other possible causes, such as chest X-rays or an echocardiogram to exclude heart failure. In this section, we'll look at three of the most common diseases that can complicate the diagnosis of asthma in adults.

The diseases formerly known as chronic bronchitis and emphysema

COPD encompasses several conditions that limit airflow, including 'chronic bronchitis' and 'emphysema'. Around 15 per cent of men and 5 per cent of women in the UK suffer from chronic bronchitis, which Bourke defines as a productive cough 'on most days for at least three months of two successive years'. Smoking or other triggers leave the airways of COPD patients inflamed and swollen, which blocks the flow of air and damages the lung. Meanwhile, goblet cells pump out more mucus. Because of the damage to the mucociliary escalator, the mucus isn't cleared, leaving a plug in the airway. The mucus is an ideal habitat for many bacteria, so COPD patients often experience regular infections (acute bronchitis).

Emphysema arises from the alveoli's gradual destruction. Alveoli and small airways depend on the support of the surrounding tissues to remain open. Emphysema destroys this support. That's one reason why the airways of people with emphysema become obstructed and collapse when they exhale. This traps air, which can stretch the lungs. Breathing using 'hyperinflated' lungs takes much more effort. Emphysema also damages other elastic tissues – such as elastin – in the lungs. As emphysema progresses, alveoli form into large, irregular pockets with holes in their walls. Not surprisingly, these changes hinder the transfer of carbon dioxide and oxygen.

Chronic obstructive pulmonary disease (COPD)

Doctors estimate that three million people in the UK suffer from COPD. Of these, two million remain undiagnosed. For example, smokers may attribute cough and phlegm to tobacco rather than COPD and so don't seek medical help. While the symptoms can seem similar, asthma essentially arises from inflamed, hyper-reactive airways. Contraction of the muscle surrounding the airways causes the obstruction, a very different process from COPD.

Traditionally, doctors have regarded asthma as reversible: in other words, attacks abate when exposure to the trigger ends or after the patient uses a bronchodilator. In contrast, they consider COPD to be largely irreversible. However, drugs can at least partially reverse the airway obstruction in many people with COPD, while remodelling (Chapter 1) can mean that people with severe asthma do not show totally reversible obstruction.

The risk factors for COPD and asthma also overlap. While smoking is the leading risk factor for COPD, many asthmatics smoke. Furthermore, bacterial infections trigger between a third and half of all COPD exacerbations, Hoshino and collaborators note. But respiratory infections are also a problem for people with asthma.

Nevertheless, COPD usually has a poorer prognosis than asthma. According to the National Institute for Health and Clinical Excellence (NICE), COPD kills approximately 30,000 people each year in the UK. According to NICE, 78 per cent of men and 72 per cent of women with mild COPD that does not require continuous drug treatment survive for a minimum of five years. But five-year survival declines to 30 and 24 per cent respectively in people with severe COPD who require oxygen or nebulized therapy (see Chapter 6).

So, it's important to get the diagnosis right (see Table 5.1 on page 69) and several clues help doctors differentiate COPD and asthma. For example:

- Asthma often has a sudden onset. COPD typically develops more gradually, typically over between 10 and 40 years, although people with sedentary lifestyles may not notice breathlessness until considerable portions of their lung function is gone.
- Asthma tends to wax and wane. While the airflow obstruction in COPD is slowly progressive, the severity does not change markedly over several months.
- Cough and sputum are more common with COPD than in asthma.
- Wheeze, a marked diurnal variation in symptoms and peak flow, and bronchial hyper-responsiveness are more common with asthma than COPD.
- Cold air is a more important trigger in asthma than COPD. Almost all asthmatics (96 per cent) show hyper-responsiveness when they inhale cold air, compared to just 10 per cent of those with COPD.

While these patterns offer important clues, doctors can't rely on a single feature to distinguish the diseases. Indeed, Dima and colleagues found that combining lung function, assessing sputum production after inhaling a saline aerosol and determining airway hyper-responsiveness helped differentiate asthma from COPD.

Against this background, NICE suggests that doctors should consider whether COPD is responsible for symptoms in those aged 35 years and over who are present or former smokers (or have another risk factor) and suffer from any of the following:

- breathlessness when they exercise;
- chronic cough;
- regular sputum production;
- frequent bouts of winter 'bronchitis';
- wheeze.

(Doctors should exclude other causes of chronic cough, including tuberculosis and bronchiectasis.)

Stanley's smoker's cough

Stanley, who's just celebrated his 68th birthday, started work at 16 years of age as an apprentice paint-sprayer in a car factory. When the site shut down, he retrained as a baker. An active trade unionist, he was well aware of the risks of occupational asthma in his previous jobs but, unlike some of his co-workers, he didn't develop symptoms. However, a few months ago, Stan sought his GP's advice as sometimes he feels breathless walking down to the local social club or working in his allotment. One of Stan's grandsons keeps nagging him to quit smoking. And even after more than half a century smoking, he wants to set a good example to his other grandchildren. 'If I can quit, they can,' he says. Stan admits to having a dreadful smoker's cough and catching 'cold after cold'. His doctor suspects COPD. But a trial of inhaled steroids and salmeterol markedly improves Stan's breathlessness and his peak flow returns to 89 per cent of his predicted level. Stanley has late-onset asthma – and he quits smoking.

Table 5.1: Features that NICE suggests may help differentiate COPD and asthma

Feature	Asthma	COPD
Smoker or ex-smoker	Possible	Nearly all
Symptoms emerged before 35 years of age	Often	Rarely
Chronic productive cough	Uncommon	Common
Breathlessness	Variable	Persistent, progressive
Night-time waking with breathlessness or wheeze	Common	Uncommon
Significant diurnal or day-to-day symtom variability	Common	Uncommon

Smoking and other causes of COPD

Smoking is the most common cause of COPD. Indeed, NICE points out, smoking causes around 85 per cent of COPD-related deaths. Furthermore, Løkke and colleagues found that at least 25 per cent of people develop moderate or severe COPD after smoking for 25 years. Indeed, 30 to 40 per cent of smokers in this study showed mild COPD or worse.

Nevertheless, some smokers never develop COPD. On the other hand, some lifelong non-smokers also suffer from COPD. Lamprecht and co-workers reported that, of people aged at least 40 years who had never smoked, 6.6 per cent suffered mild COPD and 5.6 per cent moderate to severe COPD. Indeed, people who had never smoked comprised 23.3 per cent of patients with moderate to severe COPD.

As non-smokers can develop COPD, factors other than tobacco must contribute. For instance, the immune system normally differentiates our tissue from that of invading pathogens. Occasionally, however, immunological civil war breaks out and the immune system produces antibodies against healthy tissues – so called auto-immunity. Rheumatoid arthritis, multiple sclerosis and type 1 ('juvenile') diabetes, for example, arise when autoantibodies attack joints, the fatty stealth surrounding nerve cells in the brain and the pancreas respectively. A growing body of evidence suggests that COPD patients produce autoantibodies against elastin and the cell layer lining the airways. Núñez and colleagues found abnormal levels of two antibodies linked to autoimmunity in 34 and 26 per cent of COPD patients respectively, compared to 3 and 6 per cent of controls.

Occupational COPD

Certain factors – including coalmine and silica dust, and metal fumes – can cause occupational COPD, which occasionally proves fatal. Coggon and colleagues estimated that occupational COPD accounted for approximately 172 extra deaths a year in men aged 20 to 79 years from England and Wales during 1979–90 (excluding 1981) and 83 extra deaths during 1991–2000.

Furthermore, 1 to 2 per cent of people with emphysema inherit a deficiency in a protein called alpha-1-antitrypsin (AAt), which protects the lung's elastic structures. In smokers who lack AAt, emphysema can begin in their 30s and 40s. In most smokers, emphysema begins to produce symptoms between the ages of 40 and 60 years. Nevertheless, smoking remains the most important cause of COPD (see Chapter 7 for advice on how to quit).

Heart failure and cardiac asthma

Heart failure can cause nocturnal cough and other symptoms reminiscent of asthma. During a heart attack, a blockage in blood vessels supplying the heart starves the cardiac muscle of oxygen and nutrients, and the area of the heart supplied by the blocked vessels dies. As a result, the heart pumps less effectively – a condition called heart failure.

Heart failure causes fluid to accumulate in the lungs (pulmonary oedema), which inhibits the transfer of oxygen across the thin lining of the alveoli. In some, this causes symptoms – including shortness of breath, coughing and wheezing – that are similar to asthma. While congestive heart failure commonly causes nocturnal symptoms, these tend to occur between one and two hours after lying down, rather than in the early morning as is typical of asthma. Furthermore, many people with heart failure show ankle swelling and weight gain, which are not associated with asthma.

Treatments for heart failure reduce pulmonary oedema and therefore alleviate the symptoms of cardiac asthma. But overusing asthma treatments, such as bronchodilators, can exacerbate heart failure and, because beta-agonists stimulate the heart, provoke dangerous abnormal heart rhythms. However, asthma and heart disease are common and some people develop both conditions.

Vocal cord dysfunction

In some studies, up to 40 per cent of people referred to specialists with recalcitrant asthma suffered from vocal cord dysfunction (VCD). Newman and colleagues found that 56 per cent of people hospitalized with VCD also had asthma. So 44 per cent had VCD without asthma – and VCD seems to be especially common in young women. However, doctors often confused VCD and asthma. Indeed, in patients with VCD alone, doctors misdiagnosed asthma for, on average, almost five years and 81 per cent regularly received oral steroids, which, as we'll see in the next chapter, can cause serious side effects.

VCD can hinder airflow. So, like asthma sufferers, VCD patients wheeze. However, some important clues help distinguish VCD from asthma:

- People with VCD are more likely than asthma sufferers to experience throat tightness or changes in their voice.
- Typically, people with VCD experience more problems inhaling than exhaling.
- Symptoms that are predominantly due to VCD tend to be most common during the day. Attacks tend to emerge and resolve abruptly.
- Inhaled bronchodilators have little effect, or even exacerbate, VCD.
- Patients with asthma are more likely than those with VCD to produce sputum.

6

Treating asthma in adults

During the nineteenth and early twentieth centuries, people tried a wide range of treatments including opium, morphine, caffeine and iodine to alleviate their asthma. They tried inhaling fumes from burning preparations of stramonium (derived from the hallucinogenic Jimson weed, also called thorn apple), lobelia, potash and tobacco. They even tried cauterizing (burning) the inside of their nasal passage. Some of these treatments might have helped: for example, caffeine is a chemical relative of theophylline, a drug for asthma used today. But many supposed remedies – inhaling tobacco, for example – probably made asthma worse.

The wide range of 'treatments' underscores how difficult managing asthma was before doctors started using theophylline in 1922. Salbutamol, which remains a mainstay of treatment, reached the market in 1968. A variety of bronchodilators and anti-inflammatory drugs followed, delivered by a wide range of devices. Pharmaceutical companies continue to develop new treatments for asthma, COPD and other respiratory diseases.

This wide choice of treatments and devices means that you can probably find the right combination of drugs and devices that controls your symptoms. Properly used, combining a bronchodilator ('reliever') and an anti-inflammatory ('preventer') controls most cases of asthma. And older people, despite their lower lung function (Chapter 1), find that bronchodilators and corticosteroids produce similar improvements in airways obstruction, quality of life, psychological status and disease severity as in younger people.

In this chapter, we'll look at some of the most widely used drugs and devices used to treat asthma. (As this book looks at what you can do to cope with your asthma, we won't consider the various treatments you could receive in hospital. For further information on these, try the Asthma UK and other websites listed at the end of the book.) This chapter aims to aid your discussions with GPs and asthma nurses as you work together to determine the right treatment for you.

The aims of asthma treatment

Asthma treatment aims to let you live as normal a life as possible. More specifically, doctors try to meet four aims:

- to minimize symptoms, including nocturnal and exercise-induced symptoms;
- to prevent exacerbations, and therefore minimize your need to use 'rescue' bronchodilators to alleviate asthma attacks;
- to achieve the best possible lung function – ideally to within 80 per cent of your best or predicted value.
- to minimize side effects.

Attaining these treatment goals sometimes proves more difficult in elderly asthmatics than in children or younger adults. For example, many elderly patients show some irreversible airway obstruction. So, attaining near normal lung function may be impossible or require doses of drugs that are likely to cause unacceptable side effects. On the other hand, GPs, asthma nurses and elderly asthmatics need to ensure that adults with asthma are not unnecessarily restricting their lifestyles to accommodate their symptoms.

It may be worth agreeing individual goals for you with your doctor or nurse – especially as doctors and nurses may have a different view as to what constitutes a 'good' outcome. Healthcare professionals may focus more on symptoms, while you may want to spend more time in the garden, return to work or run the London marathon. So, you need to discuss how these treatment goals can help you achieve your ambition. Minimizing exercise-induced symptoms may need more intensive therapy if you are planning to run the marathon than if you want to want to play with your kids or grandchildren in the park.

To look at the treatment goals from another angle, if you can answer yes to one or more of the following questions, you may have poorly controlled asthma and you should see your doctor or asthma nurse to review your asthma medication:

- Have you experienced difficulties sleeping because of asthma, including cough?
- Have new asthma symptoms (cough, wheeze, chest tightness or breathlessness) emerged?
- Have your usual symptoms become more severe during the day?

- Has asthma interfered with your usual activities around the home, at work or college?
- Are you using more than 10 or 12 puffs of bronchodilator a day – around two canisters a month?

Age and the response to asthma treatment

Despite the wide range of treatments, poor control remains common. Cazzoletti and colleagues found that only 15 per cent of adults who used inhaled corticosteroids during the year before the trial showed well-controlled asthma. Clatworthy and co-workers found that 38 per cent of UK patients aged between 18 and 94 years showed poorly controlled asthma. Indeed, age itself seems to make poor asthma control more likely: every additional year of age increased the chances of having poorly controlled asthma by 1 per cent. That may not sound much. But it soon adds up.

Several factors drive the increased risk of poor control as you get older. For example:

- People with adult-onset asthma may need to take higher doses of medication to maintain normal lung function, partly because their lungs are less responsive than those of younger asthmatics.
- Many adults with asthma show some degree of irreversible airway obstruction, following airway remodelling caused by inflammation and, possibly, repeated cycles of bronchoconstriction.
- Lung function seems to decline more rapidly in adults with asthma than people of the same age without asthma, again possibly because of airway remodelling.
- Older people tend to feel their symptoms are more severe than younger people do, even if their lung function tests are similar.
- Many adults may not admit that symptoms limit their activity, for example because they feel that limitations are an inevitable part of asthma or ageing. So, asthma nurses and doctors may overestimate the control produced by current treatment.

The principles of treatment

Asthma management takes, broadly, a two-pronged approach. First, inhaled corticosteroids and other anti-inflammatory drugs suppress the underlying inflammation. However, steroids dampen inflammation too slowly to relieve attacks rapidly. So, second, bronchodilators open constricted airways and alleviate exacerbations. But bronchodilators do not reduce inflammation.

Treating asthma during pregnancy

The *British Guideline* remarks that 'the risk of harm to the foetus from severe or chronically under-treated asthma outweighs any small risk from the medications used to control asthma'. For example, a large UK study found no increased risk of major congenital malformations in children born to women who used asthma treatments in the year before or during pregnancy.

You can use short-acting (relievers) and long-acting bronchodilators as normal during your pregnancy, the *British Guideline* remarks. Neither drug appears to increase the risk of major congenital malformations or other problems during pregnancy, or complications during labour and delivery. Similarly, inhaled steroids (preventers) do not seem to increase the risk of major congenital malformations or other complications. Indeed, inhaled anti-inflammatory drugs reduce the risk of suffering an exacerbation during pregnancy. As we've seen, poorly controlled asthma increases the risk of complications for mothers and babies. So, you can use inhaled steroids as usual during pregnancy. Later in this chapter, we'll look at the specific issues surrounding oral steroids in pregnancy.

In other words, most asthmatics need *both* a preventer (steroid or another anti-inflammatory) and a reliever (bronchodilator). Obviously, it's important that you don't get them confused. Read the patient information leaflet that came with the inhaler (you can obtain information about most drugs at <http://www.medicines.org.uk/emc/>) and, if you don't understand something or have a question, speak to your pharmacist, doctor or asthma nurse. It's especially important that you know how to use your inhaler correctly – as we'll see later, mistakes are common.

In the UK, doctors and nurses follow a stepped approach to treatment as laid out in the *British Guideline on the Management of Asthma* (see Figure 6.1). Doctors and nurses start treatment at the level most likely to minimize symptoms and normalize lung function, then move up to the next step if your asthma remains inadequately controlled. Once your asthma is well controlled for several months, treatment moves down a step. On the other hand, if asthma worsens, treatment can move up a step.

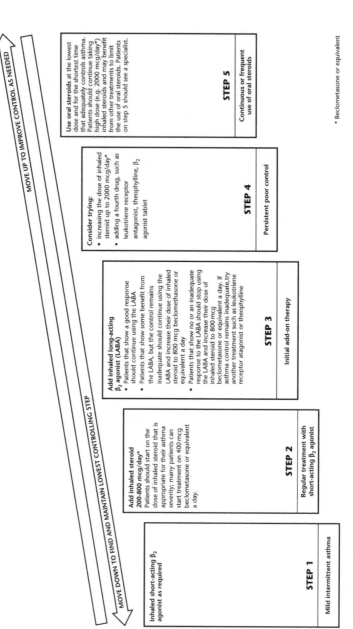

Figure 6.1 The stepped-care approach to asthma treatment advocated by and adapted from the *British Guideline on the Management of Asthma*

Self-management programmes and action plans

Self-management programmes and action plans based on the *British Guideline* put you in control of your asthma. The programmes and action plans are individualized to each patient's abilities, circumstances and understanding. Some people want as much control over their disease and treatment as possible and are willing to monitor their symptoms and peak flow rigorously. Other people would rather take a more passive role. So, it's important to be honest with your doctor or asthma nurse about how much responsibility you want. Your medical team can then develop an action plan that meets your needs.

Most self-management programmes include education about asthma and its treatment. They'll also allow you to recognize declining control based on symptoms, peak flow or both. Most summarize action to take if asthma deteriorates, including when to:

• seek emergency help;
• increase the dose of inhaled steroids;
• start oral steroids.

In the latter case, the doctor may provide you with an emergency course of steroid tablets.

Travelling with asthma

It is worth reviewing both your action plan and your treatment before you travel – especially overseas. It's better to be safe than sorry. Ensure you know when to increase your inhaled steroid dose or start oral steroids: your GP or asthma nurse won't be on the end of the phone. Make sure you also have:

• spare asthma medications (preventer and relievers);
• a short course of oral steroid (discuss taking some with you, even if you don't usually have them at home);
• adequate health insurance;
• information about local emergency and other health services in your destination;
• discussed travel vaccinations.

Flying will not affect inhalers, which you should carry and store in your hand luggage.

Receptors: unlocking your asthma

Numerous chemicals pass messages around your body:

- Hormones (such as oestrogen, testosterone and corticosteroids – see page 80) carry signals between organs, such as a gland and a fat cell or muscle.
- Mediators carry messages between cells that activate or inhibit the immune system.
- Neurotransmitters pass messages between nerves as well as between nerves and muscles. For example, the neurotransmitter noradrenaline causes the muscles around your airways to relax, and another neurotransmitter, acetylcholine, causes the same muscles to contract.

Many of these messengers bind to specific proteins, called receptors. Most receptors are on the surface of the cells where the receptor acts. However, some hormones and steroidal drugs used to treat inflammation bind to receptors inside the cell. Taking a brief look at receptors helps you understand how your asthma drugs act (see Figure 6.2).

Imagine an immune cell or a muscle cell surrounding the airway as a car. The receptor is the ignition lock. The messenger – such as an inflammatory mediator, noradrenaline or acetylcholine – is the key. When the key fits into a lock, the engine starts. And when the messenger binds to the receptor, part of the cell's internal machine switches on. So, the mediator triggers inflammation or noradrenaline induces bronchodilatation. But the effect is specific: your key only starts your car. And the message only switches on those processes controlled by the receptor. Noradrenaline doesn't bind to the receptor for acetylcholine, for example.

Now imagine you have a skeleton key. It also fits the ignition lock and switches on the engine. Some drugs – such as certain bronchodilators – act like a skeleton key. The receptor can't distinguish the drug (called an agonist) from the normal mediator. Both switch on the cell's machinery. So, a beta-agonist (a bronchodilator) has the same action as noradrenaline. (See Figure 6.2.)

Imagine you have another key. It fits the ignition lock, but won't turn so the car won't start. But while this key is in the lock, you can't get the right key in. Some drugs for asthma, such as leukotriene receptor antagonists, bind to the receptor but don't activate the internal machine (called antagonists). However, antagonists stop leukotrienes (an inflammatory mediator) from binding and promoting inflammation. So, inflammation subsides. Beta-blockers (see Chapter 2) can trigger asthma.

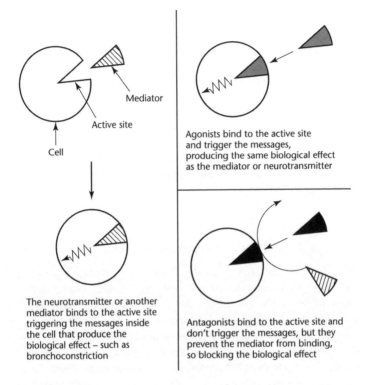

Figure 6.2 Drugs and receptors

They antagonize the same receptors that beta-agonist bronchodilators activate – and so have the opposite effect and close the airways.

Anti-inflammatory drugs

Even when you don't suffer symptoms, the inflammation that causes asthma usually remains, lurking in your lungs waiting to flare into an exacerbation. As this inflammation is chronic, you need to take your anti-inflammatory even when you feel symptom-free. Nevertheless, your doctor or asthma nurse should assess your symptoms regularly and adjust the dose of anti-inflammatory to the minimum that maintains control of your symptoms and meets the other treatment goals. This reduces the risk of side effects. Several drugs dampen asthmatic inflammation, of which steroids are the most commonly used.

Steroids

In 1930, American researchers isolated a substance, which they called cortin, from the adrenal glands (these lie on top of the kidneys). The researchers discovered that cortin contained a cocktail of hormones – corticosteroids – that have several important biological actions:

- controlling the metabolism of carbohydrates, such as starch and sugar;
- regulating the balance of minerals and electrolytes (salts) in the blood;
- regulating the amount of fluid in the body;
- reducing inflammation.

Anabolic steroids and corticosteroids

Steroids are a very large group of natural and synthetic chemicals – including corticosteroids as well as the sex hormones oestrogen, progestogen and testosterone – that produce a wide range of distinct actions. One group, called mineralocorticoids, control the body's use of minerals and electrolytes. Another group, glucocorticoids, regulate the levels of glucose in the blood. Importantly, the corticosteroids used to reduce allergic inflammation produce different effects from those produced by the 'anabolic' steroids abused by some weight-lifters, athletes and body-builders. Anabolic steroids are chemical relatives of testosterone, and are used medically to increase muscle mass and enhance physical performance. So, you won't start putting on muscle or develop other side effects linked to anabolic steroids if you take corticosteroids for asthma.

Doctors soon realized that corticosteroids could treat inflammatory diseases, so pharmaceutical companies developed synthetic steroids that reduced inflammation but produced fewer unwanted effects than the natural hormones on, for example, carbohydrate metabolism and fluid balance. Today, low-dose inhaled corticosteroids are the mainstay of asthma treatment in adults as well as children.

How corticosteroids work

As mentioned on page 78, corticosteroids cross the membrane that surrounds each cell and bind to a specific receptor. Rather like sticking two Lego bricks together, the steroid and receptor form a 'complex'. This complex moves to the nucleus, which is the cell's 'control centre'. Here, the complex binds to DNA, which contains your genetic code (Figure 6.3).

You can think of your genetic code as an instruction manual on 46 chromosomes that contains all the information needed to make you. Each gene is an instruction to make a particular protein, such as a receptor, an enzyme or a protein that maintains the body's or cell's structure.

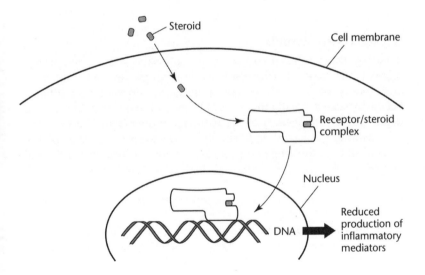

Figure 6.3 How steroids act

Almost every cell (mature red blood cells are a notable exception) contains all the DNA needed to make your entire body. (That's why you can clone an entire animal from a single cell.) But you don't need the alveoli genes to make toenails. And a particular cell doesn't need all the genes all the time. It may need some genes only when the cell needs to repair damage or divide. So, cells switch genes on and off as needed.

The steroid–receptor complex also switches certain specific genes on or off, which changes the balance of proteins produced by the cell. In particular, corticosteroids reduce production of inflammatory mediators by several types of white blood cell linked to asthma, including T cells, eosinophils and mast cells. These genetic (also called genomic) effects take several hours to emerge. Steroids also decrease the blood flow to the airways within a few minutes, which is far too quickly for steroids to change the balance of proteins in the cell by influencing genes. However, these 'non-genomic' actions are probably less important than corticosteroid's influence on gene expression in reducing the inflammation that underlies asthma.

Inhaled corticosteroids

Regularly using inhaled corticosteroids alleviates asthma symptoms, reduces the risk of exacerbations and improves lung function and quality of life. Lazarus and colleagues comment that inhaled beclomethasone usually increases FEV_1 by between 5 and 20 per cent, depending on the severity of the asthma and the extent of irreversible remodelling. So, according to the *British Guideline on the Management of Asthma*, the following groups of adults should probably use inhaled steroids:

- those who use inhaled bronchodilators three times a week or more;
- those who suffer symptoms three times a week or more;
- those who wake one or more nights a week experiencing asthmatic symptoms.

Treatment starts at a dose appropriate to the severity – often 400 mcg beclomethasone dipropionate (the most widely used inhaled steroid) per day or its equivalent (see Tables 6.1 and 6.2; a microgram [µg or mcg] is one millionth of a gram). Many adults with mild asthma find that 400 mcg a day controls their asthma. However, some people need up to 2,000 mcg beclomethasone dipropionate (or the equivalent) a day. The risk of side effects rises as the dose increases, so doctors or asthma nurses should determine the lowest dose of inhaled steroid that ensures you meet your treatment goals.

There are several steroids for asthma, administered using various delivery devices. The *British Guideline on the Management of Asthma* notes that beclomethasone dipropionate and budesonide show similar efficacy, although the potency may vary depending on the delivery device. For example, a device that creates a fine mist of very small particles will deliver a greater proportion of the dose deep into the lung than one producing larger particles.

That's why the dose of beclomethasone differs depending on whether the inhaler uses chlorofluorocarbons (CFCs) or hydrofluoroalkane (HFA) as a propellant. As CFCs damage the ozone layer, asthma devices increasingly use HFA. However, steroid particles in the HFA devices are smaller than in CFC-propelled inhalers, so the dose from some inhalers is lower.

Fluticasone and mometasone are more potent than beclomethasone and budesonide: indeed, fluticasone and mometasone need half the dose to produce the same anti-inflammatory effect. People usually, but not always, inhale these steroids twice daily. However, many asthma patients can take another steroid called ciclesonide once daily. Inhaling 160 mcg ciclesonide once daily often controls asthma. But, as with all steroids, the dose is tailored to the severity of your symptoms. In severe asthma, 320 mcg ciclesonide twice daily may reduce the frequency of exacerbations, whereas some can control their asthma with just 80 mcg once daily.

Table 6.1 Examples of low-, medium- and high-dose inhaled steroids

Steroid name	Daily dose (mcg)		
	Low	Medium	High
Beclomethasone dipropionate – CFC	200–500	500–1,000	1,000–2,000
Beclomethasone dipropionate – HFA	100–250	250–500	500–1,000
Budesonide	200–400	400–800	800–1,600
Ciclesonide	100–200	200–400	400–1,600
Fluticasone	100–250	250–500	500–1,000

Source: Based on Balter and colleagues.

Table 6.2 Examples of the equivalent doses of inhaled steroid

Steroid	Example of brands/inhaler	Equivalent dose
Beclomethasone (also spelt beclometasone)	• Clenil modulite • Clickhaler • Aerobec Autohaler • Asmabec Clickhaler • Becodisks • Easyhaler • Pulvinal • Filair	400 mcg
	• Qvar	200–300 mcg
	• Fostair	200 mcg
Budesonide	• Turbohaler • Metered-dose inhaler • Easyhaler • Novolizer • Symbicort (with formoterol)	400 mcg
Fluticasone	• Metered-dose inhaler (HFA) • Accuhaler • Seretide (with salmeterol)	200 mcg
Mometasone	Asmanex	200 mcg
Ciclesonide	Alvesco	200–300 mcg

Source: Based on the *British Guidleine on the Management of Asthma.*

Side effects of inhaled steroids

Inhaled steroids are, generally, relatively safe and less hazardous to your health than poorly controlled asthma. Nevertheless, inhaled steroids can cause several adverse events. For example, according to the *British Guideline*, in adults doses of less than 800 mcg beclometasone dipropionate per day (or equivalent) can cause oral thrush (oral candidiasis) and dysphonia:

• *Oral candidiasis*: Oral candidiasis (thrush in the mouth) is the most common fungal infection among humans. Between 20 and 75 per cent of humans carry members of the candida family in our mouths, Akpan and Morgan point out. Our immune systems usually prevent the fungi from spreading and causing symptoms. However, inhaled steroids can suppress the mouth's immune defences. This allows candida to grow, forming white patches around the gums, palates and tongue. Indeed, up to one in 20 people taking inhaled corticosteroids develop oral candidiasis. You can reduce the risk by rinsing and spitting after inhaling the steroid or by using a spacer (see page 101).

- *Dysphonia*: Dysphonia refers to changes in your voice's ability to make sounds. Almost everyone has suffered laryngitis (inflammation of the voice box) following an infection – it can make your voice sound hoarse, weak, harsh or rough. (Think of the last time you had a 'frog in your throat'.) And between 2 and 6 per cent of people taking inhaled steroids develop dysphonia. Higher doses of inhaled steroids are especially likely to cause dysphonia.

Skin side effects

Steroids can 'thin the skin' (atrophy) by removing protein. They can also produce red or purple discolorations, called purpura, caused by blood vessels leaking near the skin's surface. Because of this skin thinning, inhaled steroids may mean you bruise easily, especially if you're older, taking higher doses of steroid or using long-term treatment.

The forearms and lower legs seem to be especially prone to steroid-related bruising. This pattern led some researchers to suggest that ultraviolet light interacted with the steroid to cause skin atrophy. Using moisturizers and protecting your skin from sunlight (e.g. with sunscreen) may help protect against bruising.

Steroids can also trigger a sudden outbreak of acne in adults, typically those aged 35 to 75 years. The acne tends to be worse on the trunk than on other parts of the body. In other cases, inhaled steroids taken long term can cause fine downy hair to appear on the sides of the face, upper lip and chin (hirsutism). Skin thinning, acne and hirsutism are more common with oral than inhaled steroids. Nevertheless, these side effects occur occasionally in people taking inhaled steroids, especially at high doses.

Diabetes

Doctors realized many years ago that oral steroids potentially trigger diabetes. However, more recent studies suggest that inhaled steroids, especially at high doses, may also cause diabetes. For example, Suissa and collaborators followed 388,584 adults using inhaled corticosteroids for asthma or COPD for, on average, 5.5 years. Over this time, inhaled corticosteroids increased the risk of developing diabetes by 34 per cent. Inhaled corticosteroids also increased the likelihood that people with diabetes would progress from oral hypoglycaemic (blood-sugar lowering) agents to insulin (suggesting that their diabetes got worse) by 34 per cent.

The risk rose progressively with increasing steroid doses. Compared to people not using inhaled corticosteroids, the risk of developing diabetes for the first time increased from 18 per cent with low-dose steroids (less than 500 mcg fluticasone or equivalent daily) to 30 per cent with moderate doses (500–999 mcg or equivalent daily). The increased risk reached 64 per cent with high doses (at least 1,000 mcg fluticasone or equivalent daily). Similarly, the risk of progressing from oral hypoglycaemic agents to insulin increased from 8 per cent with low doses to 30 and 54 per cent with moderate and high doses respectively.

Other serious side-effects

Other serious side effects – including changes in bone density, cataracts and glaucoma – occur in less than 1 per cent of people using inhaled steroids. Again, these side effects generally emerge only at higher doses, during prolonged treatment or both, and are much more common with oral than inhaled steroids (see page 87). For example, when doctors analysed the scientific studies, beclometasone dipropionate did not seem to influence bone density at doses up to 1,000 mcg. (Bone density measures the strength of your skeleton. Low density means a weak skeleton and therefore a greater risk of suffering a broken bone.)

When to increase your dose of steroid

If you don't meet the goals of treatment or experience an exacerbation, your GP or asthma nurse might suggest that you increase your dose of steroid or add another drug to your daily treatment (see page 76). But before you increase your dose of steroid or start a new drug, there are certain checks you and your healthcare professionals should make:

- Have you taken your existing drugs as prescribed? Clatworthy and colleagues found that poor adherence to inhaled steroids increased the risk of poor asthma control by 35 per cent.
- Is your inhaler technique correct? (We'll return to this later in the chapter.)
- As far as possible, have you eliminated or treated trigger factors, such as smoking, allergens and rhinitis (e.g. hay fever)? Clatworthy and colleagues found that rhinitis increased the risk of poorly controlled asthma almost five-fold, and smoking around four-fold. Even in people with mild asthma, Lazarus and co-authors comment, smoking blunts the response to inhaled corticosteroids. So, people who smoke may need higher doses of inhaled steroids than non-smokers.
- Do you need to check whether the diagnosis is correct or whether

you've developed a concurrent disease that reduces the effectiveness of treatment? For example, anti-inflammatory therapy may have a less marked benefit in people with both asthma and COPD compared to those with asthma alone.

In most patients, doubling the dose of inhaled corticosteroids does not halve the severity of asthma symptoms. The severity may decline by only a third or a quarter, for example. (Researchers describe this as a flat dose-response curve.) However, some patients benefit more than others from higher doses of inhaled corticosteroids. Unfortunately, doctors cannot tell who will benefit from higher doses in advance so, rather than increasing the dose of steroid, your GP or nurse may suggest adding in another drug (usually a long-acting bronchodilator). But if 800 mcg beclometasone dipropionate a day or equivalent plus a long-acting bronchodilator or another add-in therapy still fails to control your symptoms adequately, the *British Guideline on the Management of Asthma* suggests increasing the steroid dose to up to 2,000 mcg a day.

Oral steroids

Inhaled steroids control most cases of asthma. However, if your asthma remains difficult to control, or you suffer a severe exacerbation or show a potentially dangerous decline in lung function, your doctor may prescribe a course of steroid tablets, usually prednisolone, generally lasting a week or two. Very few asthma patients take oral steroids regularly.

The dose delivered by oral steroids is much higher than the inhaled counterparts, so oral steroids are highly effective at controlling the inflammation underlying asthma and can be lifesavers. However, the risk of developing side effects is much greater with oral than inhaled steroids. Some side effects emerge rapidly, such as mood changes (like feeling anxious, irritable, depressed or 'high') and stomach problems. Others – such as weakness or a rounder face – take several weeks or months, or a number of courses, to emerge. Elderly asthmatics may be especially prone to these side effects, as they often metabolize (break down) steroids less rapidly than younger patients.

The *British Guideline on the Management of Asthma* notes that those taking steroid tablets long term (for example, for more than three months) or requiring frequent courses (such as three to four or more times a year) are at risk of potentially serious side effects. So, doctors or nurses should regularly check:

- blood pressure and cholesterol levels, to monitor the risk of heart disease;
- levels of sugar in urine or blood, to check for diabetes;

- bone mineral density, to watch for osteoporosis (brittle bone disease);
- eyes, for cataracts (clouding of the lens).

Many of the common side effects with oral steroids (which we'll discuss in a moment) are dose-related. We've already discussed some of these side effects (such as skin thinning, acne and hirsutism) with inhaled steroids, but the risk is markedly higher with oral steroids.

Furthermore, your body can adapt to oral steroids. So, stopping long-term treatment abruptly can trigger withdrawal reactions, including muscle and joint pain, conjunctivitis, fever, weight loss, runny nose and painful, itchy skin lumps. You should always seek advice from a doctor or asthma nurse before stopping, or reducing the dose of, oral steroids.

Oral steroids and infections

If you have never suffered from chicken pox or shingles, you need to stay away from people with these infections. Oral steroids suppress the immune response. As a result, *Varicella zoster* virus, which is responsible for chicken pox and shingles, can cause serious complications (including pneumonia) and even prove fatal in people taking oral steroids. If you encounter anyone suffering from chicken pox or shingles you should see your GP immediately. Long-term treatment with oral steroids can exacerbate other diseases or lead to unusual symptoms. So, if you feel unwell it is especially important to seek your doctor's advice.

Osteoporosis and bone loss

Approximately three million people in the UK have osteoporosis, which causes more than 230,000 fractured bones every year. Osteoporosis is common in post-menopausal women. However, steroids can cause osteoporosis as well as exacerbating the 'natural' age-related decline in skeletal strength. Oral steroids can also cause muscle wasting and weakness – especially in the back, hips, ribs and arms – and unusual tiredness. These changes may increase the risk of a fall – and, therefore, the risk that you will break a bone, especially if your skeleton is already brittle.

Despite appearances, your skeleton isn't inert. The stresses and strains of daily life create numerous tiny cracks in your bones, which would eventually undermine your skeleton's strength. To prevent this, a group of cells called osteoclasts break down old bone by creating microscopic pits on the skeleton's surface. Another group of cells, the osteoblasts, fill in the pits with new bone. This maintains your skeleton's strength (bone mineral density, to use the technical term). However, oral steroids seem to reduce bone mineral density by, for example, reducing the amount of calcium absorbed from the diet, suppressing the formation of osteoblasts and killing osteoclasts.

Taking 5 mg prednisolone or more (or equivalent) each day decreases bone mineral density and therefore increases fracture risk, irrespective of age or sex. For example, after taking oral steroids for three to six months your risk of suffering a broken hip almost doubles. Meanwhile, the chance of experiencing a vertebral (spinal) fracture almost trebles and the risk of breaking a forearm rises by around 10 per cent.

The risk of suffering a fracture declines after you stop taking oral steroids. Dore remarks that around two years after stopping oral steroids, the risk of suffering a fracture is the about the same as that in someone who has never taken these drugs. In general, inhaled steroids do not affect bone, although high doses (more than 2,000 µg/day beclomethasone or equivalent) taken for several years may cause osteoporosis.

To reduce the risk of fracture, you should take the lowest dose of inhaled and oral steroid that controls your asthma symptoms, for the shortest possible time. (But because of the risk of provoking an asthma attack or suffering withdrawal symptoms, don't stop taking your steroid or change the dose without talking to your doctor or nurse first.) Dore also suggests protecting your skeleton with exercise and ensuring you get enough calcium (1,000 to 1,500 mg per day) and vitamin D (800 to 1,000 IU per day), which may mean taking a supplement; a pint of milk contains about 750 mg of calcium, for example. Doctors can prescribe medicines that treat osteoporosis.

Cataracts and other eye problems

The transparent lens at the front of your eye focuses light on the sensitive retina that lines the rear of your eyeball. Cataracts are cloudy patches in the lens. As cataracts reduce the amount of light that reaches the retina, your vision may become blurred or cloudy. Eventually, untreated cataracts can cause blindness.

Even in people who are not taking steroids, cataracts become increasingly common with advancing age. Indeed, at least half of all people over the age of 65 years in the UK have some cataract in one or both eyes. But inhaled and oral steroids seem to increase the risk of developing cataracts, in part, Gibson and colleagues remark, by disrupting the normal turnover of cells that keeps the lens clear. In addition, oral steroids can cause glaucoma. Again, this can, if untreated, damage the nerves that carry signals from the retina to the brain, leading to loss of vision.

All adults should have their eyes checked regularly; an eye test can detect diseases such as glaucoma and cataracts before they affect your vision. But regular checks are especially important for people taking oral steroids.

Skin problems and hormonal changes

As mentioned earlier, steroids remove protein from the skin, causing skin thinning, reddish or purple 'stretch marks' (striae) in the skin, unusual bruising and wounds that won't heal. Steroids can also alter the production of hormones by the body, such as suppressing the adrenal gland. The changes to hormone levels can increase the amount of fat in the face and shoulders – known as 'moon face' and 'buffalo hump' respectively. Women taking oral steroids may find their periods become irregular or stop.

While these side effects are unpleasant, you need to remember that oral steroids could save your life. So, make sure you follow your regular treatment course, monitor your symptoms and tackle any trigger factors. This should reduce the likelihood that you'll need a course of oral steroids. But if and when you do need oral steroids, you should take them as prescribed. You might want to discuss the risks and benefits with your doctor or asthma nurse before you need to resort to the tablets.

Oral steroids during pregnancy

In general, steroid tablets do not appear to cause birth defects. However, some studies suggest that oral steroids may slightly increase the risk of cleft palate or lips, especially if used during the first trimester. The *British Guideline* comments that the association between steroid tablets and oral clefts is 'not definite and even if it is real, the benefit to the mother and the fetus of steroids for treating a life threatening disease justify the use of steroids in pregnancy'.

Some studies suggest that expectant mothers who take steroid tablets are more likely to develop pregnancy-induced hypertension (pre-eclampsia) or premature labour, while the growth of the developing baby may be impaired. In one study, oral steroids reduced the length of pregnancy by, on average, about 15 days. In many cases, however, severe asthma – which can also cause these problems – makes it difficult to tease cause from effect.

The *British Guideline* notes that pregnant women with severe asthma should use steroid tablets as and when they're required. Doctors and asthma nurses should fully discuss the reasons why, for most women who need oral steroids, the benefits outweigh the risks. So, if you're worried about the risk, speak to your doctor or asthma nurse.

Non-steroid anti-inflammatories

Sodium cromoglicate and nedocromil

Healers in the Middle East have traditionally used the plant khella (*Ammi visnaga*) – a member of the same botanical family as carrots, celery and parsnip – to treat renal colic (pain in and around the kidneys, often caused by stones). The dried flower stalks made useful toothpicks. Between the 1940s and 1960s, researchers prepared thousands of chemical variations on khella's active ingredients. Doctors started using one of these – sodium cromoglicate – in 1967 to treat asthma. Sodium cromoglicate (also spelt cromoglycate) and a related drug called nedocromil stabilize mast cells, making these important immune cells (see Chapter 1) less likely to release their stores of inflammatory mediators.

However, as they work on only a single type of cell, sodium cromoglicate and nedocromil are generally less effective than inhaled steroids at controlling asthma. Furthermore, most studies assessing sodium cromoglicate and nedocromil treated younger patients suffering from allergic asthma rather than older adults with intrinsic asthma. Nevertheless, sodium cromoglicate and nedocromil can be valuable treatments for people who cannot or won't take inhaled steroids or for some cases of exercise-induced asthma.

Leukotriene receptor antagonists

In 1938, scientists found that injecting cobra venom into the lungs of guinea pigs triggers bronchoconstriction. At the time, biologists believed that histamine caused bronchoconstriction. But antihistamines did not block the venom's effect, suggesting another substance was responsible. In 1979, researchers finally discovered that mast cells released the 'mystery mediators' – a group of three related chemicals called leukotrienes.

Since then, biologists have identified several types of leukotriene. One group of these mediators, produced by several inflammatory cells (including eosinophils, basophils and mast cells), is called the cysteinyl leukotrienes and contributes to asthma in several ways:

- by increasing the permeability (leakiness) of, and dilating, blood vessels in the lung;
- by contracting the rings of muscle surrounding the airways, causing bronchoconstriction;
- by increasing mucus secretion and impairing mucociliary clearance.

Indeed, levels of cysteinyl leukotrienes in the lung rise as asthma becomes more severe.

The link between these mediators and asthma suggests that leukotriene receptor antagonists (such as montelukast and zafirlukast) may be a logical approach to controlling asthmatic inflammation. As a rule of thumb, leukotriene receptor antagonists produce a similar improvement in lung function and bronchial hyper-responsiveness as 400 mcg beclomethasone. However, Nyenhuis and colleagues point out, older adults may produce less cysteinyl leukotrienes than younger people. This may undermine the effectiveness of leukotriene receptor antagonists in older people. So, doctors and nurses tend to add leukotriene receptor antagonists to inhaled corticosteroids. The combination controls inflammation more effectively than either drug used alone.

Certain people seem to benefit particularly from using a leukotriene receptor antagonist:

- those with marked inflammation in their upper airways (for example, caused by allergic rhinitis or nasal polyps);
- people with aspirin-sensitive asthma;
- people who experience marked exercise-induced bronchoconstriction;
- people who experience problems using inhalers – montelukast and zafirlukast are tablets.

Nevertheless, doctors can't predict with certainty who will benefit more from adding a leukotriene receptor antagonist rather than a long-acting beta-agonist (see page 96) to the steroid, so your doctor or nurse will probably offer you a trial with leukotriene receptor antagonist. If symptoms haven't improved after between four and six weeks' treatment, it's worth discussing an alternative. Patients commonly switch from a leukotriene receptor antagonist to a long-acting beta-agonist, or vice versa, if the initial choice does not adequately control symptoms.

Theophylline

Theophylline is a member of a family of chemicals – called xanthenes – that includes caffeine. Indeed, tea contains small amounts of theophylline, the first modern asthma drug. Doctors started treating asthma with theophylline in 1922.

Theophylline, which is a tablet rather than inhaled, relaxes the muscles surrounding the airways and therefore acts as a bronchodilator. It also loosens bronchial mucus, which unblocks the airways, and inhibits T-lymphocytes, a type of white blood cell involved in allergic asthma (see page 21). However, theophylline is not an especially potent anti-inflammatory, at least compared to inhaled steroids.

Theophylline works by blocking an enzyme, phosphodiesterase.

A complex array of chemical networks carries messages around the inside of our cells. One of phosphodiesterase's actions is to control the duration of these messages. Different cells use different types of phosphodiesterases. Many inflammatory cells produce a type called phosphodiesterase 4 (PDE4). Theophylline is relatively non-selective, acting on several types of phosphodiesterase. But drugs targeting PDE4 selectively are now used to treat COPD and, in the Far East, asthma.

Unfortunately, a relatively small difference separates the dose of theophylline that alleviates asthma and that causing unacceptable side effects, such as abdominal pain, diarrhoea, headache, rapid heartbeat (tachycardia), palpitations and abnormal heart rhythm (arrhythmias), insomnia, nausea, nervousness, tremor, vomiting and liver disease. Indeed, in some patients the beneficial and 'toxic' doses overlap, and older people seem to be particularly sensitive to theophylline's side effects.

This risk of side effects means that the dose of theophylline needs to be carefully tailored for each person. In many cases, this means regular blood tests to measure levels of the drug, especially as numerous factors can influence the way the body breaks down (metabolizes) theophylline. For example, smoking and heavy alcohol use can lower levels, reducing theophylline's efficacy. Viral infections, heart failure and liver disease can increase levels, potentially causing side effects.

Numerous drugs that you may take for a concurrent condition can also influence theophylline levels. For instance, cimetidine (used to treat indigestion and stomach ulcers) and the antibiotics ciprofloxacin and erythromycin can reduce theophylline's breakdown by enzymes in the liver, causing blood levels to rise to toxic concentrations. This means that you must make sure your doctor and pharmacist know you're taking theophylline when you are prescribed a new drug or buy a medicine over the counter. You should also tell your doctor or pharmacist if you are using herbal medicines or another complementary therapy. Again, some of these can interact with theophylline (or, for that matter, several other drugs used to treat other ailments).

Finally, different brands may release different doses of theophylline. Check that the pharmacist gives you the exact brand that you have been prescribed. You should change brand only after discussing the switch with your doctor or asthma nurse. Because of these problems, doctors tend to use theophylline only when long-acting beta-agonist (see p. 96) and leukotriene receptor antagonists have failed to adequately control symptoms.

Omalizumab

Antibodies are exquisitely sensitive, able to pick the proverbial molecular needle from the surrounding cellular haystack. So, researchers can use antibodies to tease apart the pathways that lead to asthma or other diseases: the antibody can switch off a particular protein, for example. This specific action also means that antibodies can treat serious diseases such as cancer, arthritis and other inflammatory diseases, including asthma. You can also set an antibody to catch an antibody. Omalizumab is an antibody that stops IgE from binding to its receptors on mast cells and basophils, so preventing the release of inflammatory mediators triggered by the allergen.

Omalizumab is added to the current treatment of adults and adolescents (12 years and older) who have unstable severe asthma despite optimized standard therapy. You receive shots of omalizumab every two to four weeks. Doctors prescribe omalizumab only when you've received full trial of, and have complied with, inhaled high-dose corticosteroids, long-acting beta-agonists and, when appropriate, leukotriene receptor antagonists, theophylline, oral corticosteroids, bronchodilator tablets and smoking cessation. Furthermore, doctors need to confirm that you produce IgE to a perennial allergen, and to establish that this has caused the unstable disease. By 'unstable', doctors mean, for example, that you have:

- experienced at least two severe exacerbations of asthma that required hospital admission within the previous year;
- suffered at least three severe exacerbations within the previous year, at least one of which required hospital admission, and a further two that required treatment or monitoring in addition to the usual care, in an A&E department.

Omalizumab's most common adverse events, NICE notes, are bruising, redness and pain at the injection site. However, omalizumab can also cause severe allergic reactions (anaphylaxis), such as bronchospasm, hypotension (dangerously low blood pressure), syncope (fainting), urticaria (a skin reaction also called 'hives') and angioedema (serious swelling) of the throat or tongue. Anaphylaxis can occur after the first dose but has been known to develop after a year's treatment. Because of the risk of anaphylaxis, omalizumab is administered only under a doctor's or nurse's supervision and you'll be monitored carefully. Patients who don't show an adequate response after 16 weeks' treatment don't receive further courses.

The last resort

As a last resort, specialists may try a short course of potent immuno-suppressants, such as methotrexate, ciclosporin (also spelt cyclosporine) and oral gold. These drugs are more commonly used to treat other inflammatory conditions – doctors prescribe methotrexate and oral gold for rheumatoid arthritis, for example, and ciclosporin, among other uses, prevents the body from rejecting transplanted organs. While immunosuppressants decrease a person's need to take oral steroids long term, they have potentially serious side effects. Fortunately, few patients need to take these drugs of last resort.

Bronchodilators

Bronchodilators relax the ring of muscle surrounding the airways, so the airway opens (dilates). Two types of bronchodilators are used to treat asthma:

- Short-acting bronchodilators ('relievers') ease breathlessness during asthma attacks and can prevent exercise-induced symptoms.
- Long-acting bronchodilators (sometimes called long-acting beta-agonists) are taken in addition to anti-inflammatory drugs if you don't meet your treatment goals with inhaled steroids alone.

Bronchodilators do not reduce the inflammation that underlies asthma, so you still need to take your anti-inflammatory regularly.

Short-acting bronchodilators

Short-acting bronchodilators ('relievers') – such as salbutamol and terbutaline – stimulate beta-receptors (see p. 50) in the ring of muscle that surrounds the airways. So, they're also called beta-agonists or β_2-agonists. (They act on one specific subtype – the $beta_2$-receptor.) Several different inhalers can deliver short-acting beta-agonists, including Accuhaler, Clickhaler and Turbohaler, so you should be able to find one that you can use. (We'll look at the different types of inhaler later in the chapter.)

The dilation of bronchi produced by short-acting beta-agonists peaks within 15 minutes and lasts between four and six hours. This pattern of activity makes short-acting beta-agonists highly effective at treating asthma attacks as well as preventing exercise-induced exacerbations. Indeed, according to the *British Guideline on the Management of Asthma*, people who experience asthma symptoms even occasionally should receive a short-acting beta-agonist.

As asthma attacks can be unpredictable, you should make sure that you always carry your bronchodilator with you. However, don't over-rely on the reliever: overuse may disguise the severity of the underlying disease. It's a bit like papering over the cracks on a wall. Sooner or later the inflammation will break through, possibly triggering a severe attack.

Keeping a note of how much you use short-acting bronchodilators can help you track whether your asthma is well controlled. If it is, you'll probably have little need to resort to short-acting bronchodilators. On the other hand, using two or more canisters of beta-agonists per month, or taking more than 10–12 puffs per day, may suggest that your asthma is poorly controlled – and you may be at risk of suffering a fatal or near-fatal attack. So, ask your doctor or asthma nurse to review your treatment.

Few people develop short-acting beta-agonists' side effects – which include tremor, palpitations and muscle cramps – unless they use high doses. If you feel that your short-acting inhaler is producing side effects, you should speak to your asthma nurse or GP. Suffering side effects may suggest that you're using too much beta-agonist and you need to change the dose of anti-inflammatory.

Long-acting beta$_2$-agonists

As we've seen, drugs such as salbutamol dilate bronchi for between four and six hours. Another group of drugs, the long-acting beta$_2$-agonists (LABA), keep the bronchi open for at least 12 hours. So, if you take them twice daily, LABAs keep the airways open throughout the day and night. Despite their effectiveness, you must always take LABAs alongside, and not instead of, anti-inflammatory drugs.

If low-dose inhaled corticosteroids don't control your symptoms adequately, your doctor or nurse may suggest combination therapy with a LABA. According to the *British Guideline*, several studies suggest that adding a LABA to low-dose inhaled corticosteroids (200–800 mcg beclometasone dipropionate a day or equivalent) reduces the number of exacerbations, decreases the need for reliever medication, alleviates nocturnal symptoms and improves quality of life more effectively than doubling the steroid dose.

However, not everyone's symptoms improve adequately after starting a LABA – some respond better to a leukotriene receptor antagonist (see page 91). Your doctor or asthma nurse may suggest that you try the LABA and see whether your symptoms improve. The length of a trial depends on your main symptom: a trial lasting days or weeks may be enough to assess if nocturnal awakenings improve, while preventing exacerbations or decreasing the use of oral steroids may require weeks or months.

Currently, doctors can chose between two LABAs, formoterol and salmeterol, which work in slightly different ways. In general, drugs act by binding to a relatively small region on the receptor called the active site. This is rather like the keyhole in a large lock. Salmeterol has a 'head' that binds to the active site and relaxes the muscle. A long tail flows behind the head, and the end of this tail sticks to another part of the receptor – equivalent to the metal plate surrounding the keyhole. Conventional beta-agonists 'drift away' from the active site after binding (one reason why they're short-acting). However, the tail means that salmeterol's head continually 'bounces' in and out of contact with the active site. This keeps the receptor stimulated and the airways open.

Formoterol acts in a different way. The drug deposits in the fatty membrane that surrounds each cell in the lung. When drug levels in the surrounding tissue fall, formoterol leaches from the membrane and stimulates the receptor. Formoterol works more rapidly than salmeterol, dilating airways within one to three minutes while salmeterol's maximum effects take around 20 minutes to emerge. This allows some people to use formoterol to alleviate asthma attacks – but talk it over with your GP or asthma nurse first.

Salmeterol mildly inhibits the release of inflammatory mediators from mast cells, but this is not effective enough to replace other anti-inflammatory drugs. So, you should only use LABAs if you are already taking inhaled corticosteroids. Indeed, LABAs are now available combined with steroids in a single inhaler. There's no difference in efficacy compared to using two inhalers, each containing a single drug. But the single inhaler guarantees that you don't forget to take the inhaled steroid with the LABA.

Oral beta-agonists

Apart from inhaling bronchodilators, you can take beta-agonists as tablets, capsules or syrups. For example, the body breaks bambuterol down to release the active ingredient, terbutaline. Other oral broncho-dilator formulations contain salbutamol. The tablets slowly release the beta-agonist, producing sustained bronchodilatation. You'll need to take your steroid as regularly as you would with an inhaled LABA.

Short-acting oral formulations – such as terbutaline and salbutamol syrups and immediate-release tablets – offer a 'reliever' for people unable to use an inhaler (perhaps because they are physically impaired). However, oral beta-agonists often produce more side effects than their inhaled counterparts.

Antimuscarinics

Two sets of nerves control the muscles that surround the airways. Adrenergic nerves act through beta-receptors to dilate the airways when your body needs more oxygen. However, you don't need your airways fully open all the time: airways also need to constrict to protect your delicate lungs from damage from cold air, pollution and so on.

Branches from another nerve – the vagus – contract airways by releasing a transmitter called acetylcholine that binds to muscarinic receptors. So, if you block (antagonize) acetylcholine, the airways will open. Another group of bronchodilators, the antimuscarinics (such as ipratropium), work in this way. They bind to, but don't activate, muscarinic receptors. But as they've stuck to the receptor, acetylcholine cannot bind – which produces bronchodilatation.

Antimuscarinics (also called anticholinergics) act more slowly than beta-agonists, taking about an hour to reach the maximum broncho-dilation. The bronchodilatation lasts for around four to six hours. This slow onset makes antimuscarinics less effective than beta-agonists for exacerbations, which need rapid relief. Indeed, most people with asthma find the bronchodilatation produced by antimuscarinics is less marked than that following beta-agonists.

On the other hand, antimuscarinics may be less likely to cause tremor and arrhythmias than beta-agonists and may be useful if people have certain cardiovascular conditions. They are also widely used to treat COPD. Some people with asthma who also develop COPD tend to use high bronchodilator doses, and these people may benefit from using ipratropium relatively early in their course of treatment.

Stepping down treatment

As we've seen, your GP or asthma nurse will advise you to increase the dose and number of drugs until your symptoms are well controlled and you've reached your treatment goals. However, the symptoms of asthma usually wax and wane – if, for example, exposure to the allergen changes or your fitness level improves. Furthermore, once the underlying inflammation is well controlled, you need lower doses of steroid to keep your asthma at bay.

As a result, the *British Guideline on the Management of Asthma* emphasizes the importance of stepping down therapy once asthma has been well controlled for a reasonable time. However, the *Guideline* notes, the step-down stage is 'often not implemented' – in other words, doctors and asthma nurses move patients up the steps but don't reduce the intensity of treatment as readily. So, some patients are over-treated, leaving them at risk of unnecessary side effects.

The *Guideline* suggests that adults who have reached their treatment goals and whose asthma has remained stable for at least three months could decrease their dose of inhaled steroid by approximately 25–50 per cent. If you feel your asthma has been stable for three months or more, talk to your doctor or asthma nurse about reducing your dose.

You'll need to monitor your lung function and symptoms carefully.

Overall, you should aim to use the lowest possible dose of inhaled steroid that adequately controls your symptoms. Nevertheless, you may need to be prepared (for instance, using a self-management plan) to step up treatment again if or when symptoms re-emerge.

Inhaler devices

Numerous inhalers can deliver anti-inflammatories and bronchodilators, so you should be able to find a device that suits you and that you can use without making critical mistakes.

Unfortunately several factors may hinder adults' ability to use inhalers, including poor vision, loss of fine motor control and weak inhalation. In one study, Gibson and co-authors remark, 10–15 per cent of people aged 20 to 40 years made a mistake using their dry powder inhaler (DPI; see page 100) that affected the amount of drug they inhaled. The proportion making a mistake increased to 40 and 60 per cent among those aged more than 60 and 80 years respectively.

The technique varies between inhalers, so always read the educational materials in the pack carefully and – importantly – ask your doctor or nurse to demonstrate. (You can check the patient information at <http:// www.medicines.org.uk/emc/>.) You can also find videos showing how to use some inhalers on the net, including on Asthma UK's site (for details see page 122). Your doctor or nurse should regularly check your inhaler technique: it's easy to slip into bad habits. If this hasn't been done for a while, you could ask a healthcare professional to make sure your technique remains adequate.

Certainly, training seems to increase the likelihood you'll use the inhaler correctly. Brocklebank and colleagues reviewed studies examining how well people used their inhaler. They found that between 23 and 43 per cent of patients got all steps correct when using a metered dose inhaler (MDI; see next section). Between 55 and 57 per cent of those using a spacer with an MDI performed all the steps correctly, compared to 53–59 per cent with a DPI. After training, 63 per cent of those using MDIs and 65 per cent of those using DPIs performed all the steps correctly.

Metered dose inhalers

MDIs, which reached the market in 1956, remain the most widely used device in asthma management. Basically, you press on the canister that contains the drug ('actuation') while breathing in slowly and steadily. You need to continue to breathe in after the inhaler has delivered the drug payload to make sure the medicine reaches as much of your airways as possible. You should then hold your breath for ten seconds.

While many people can use MDIs, these have certain limitations. For example, some people find timing the inhalation while spraying the medication difficult, although the newer MDIs that use HFA as a propellant are often easier to use than the older CFC-driven devices.

Furthermore, some of propellant remains in the MDI canister after you have used all the drug, so it can also be difficult to know when you need to replace your inhaler. You could note when you should replace your inhaler in your diary. (This is especially important with steroids. After all, you'll soon know if the bronchodilator doesn't improve your breathlessness during an attack.) Check the insert for the number of doses, then divide by the number of puffs each day; or ask your GP, asthma nurse or pharmacist for advice on when you should ask for a repeat prescription.

Only between 10 and 20 per cent of the dose of drug inhaled from an MDI reaches the lower airways. The rest deposits in the mouth and throat and is swallowed. The drug moves from the gut into blood vessels supplying the liver, which then breaks down most of the steroid or beta-agonist that you absorb in this way. Only a tiny amount of the drug you swallow reaches the general circulation. Nevertheless, even this small amount can cause side effects, especially if you take large doses.

Breath-actuated inhalers and dry powder inhalers

Most people can learn to use MDIs, but those who have trouble inhaling from an MDI may find alternative devices easier to use. Often, these newer inhalers include a counter or let you see when you're reaching the end of the drug supply.

Breath-actuated inhalers (such as the Autohaler and the Easibreathe) do away with the need to co-ordinate actuation and inhalation. The valve on the inhaler opens only when you inhale. But you still need to breathe in slowly and deeply, as well as hold your breath after the device delivers the drug.

Dry powder inhalers (such as the Turbohaler, Diskhaler, Accuhaler and Clickhaler) don't use a propellant. The force of the airflow as you inhale releases the powered drug, so you don't need to co-ordinate actuation and inspiration. However, you need to be able to generate an adequate airflow when you breathe in. In many cases, you may need to generate more inspiratory force than with an MDI. And some (but not all) DPIs need manual dexterity to use, making them less suitable for some elderly people and other adults with weaknesses due to nerve or muscle problems, or suffering from arthritis and other physical impairments.

Spacers

Spacers increase the amount of drug that reaches the airways, make MDIs easier to use, and so improve effectiveness and reduce the risk of side effects. For example:

- Large-volume spacers (e.g. Volumatic and Aerochamber) roughly double the amount of steroid that reaches the lower airway compared to an MDI used alone. Indeed, using a spacer may mean that you can use a lower total dose of steroid.
- Spacers reduce the amount of steroid deposited in the back of the mouth and throat, which reduces the risk of dysphonia and oral candidiasis.
- Spacers can help reduce the need to co-ordinate actuation (pressing the inhaler) and inhalation when using an MDI.

You place the MDI in one end of the spacer and breathe through the mouthpiece. A one-way valve closes when you exhale. The distance results in a plume of fine particles and makes co-ordinating actuation and inhalation easier. You should clean the spacer monthly in detergent and ask your doctor or asthma nurse for a replacement every year.

Nebulizers

Nebulizers force oxygen or compressed air through a small hole. This creates a change in pressure that draws the drug solution into the airstream. The airstream strikes a small sphere, forming an aerosol of small particles carrying the drug, which you inhale using a mask or mouthpiece. Larger droplets hit the wall and fall back into the solution.

Nebulizers effectively deliver high doses of bronchodilator during an acute asthma attack. Some people keep nebulizers at home if, for example, they suffer regular serious exacerbations. But you still need to take your anti-inflammatory regularly, and don't delay seeking urgent medical advice during severe acute attacks.

Nebulizers can also deliver steroids. However, properly used DPIs and MDIs used with a spacer deliver a greater proportion of the drug into the airway than nebulizers. As a result, nebulizers tend to be used to deliver steroids only if people can't use conventional inhalers.

Anne's asthma – and her arthritis

Anne – a 68-year-old retired teacher – finds her asthma is getting worse; she's waking up on more nights and feels breathless after walking her dog. But she's more worried about the pain in her hands. Over the last year or so, osteoarthritis made it increasingly difficult for her to knit and write. She's even beginning to have trouble turning the key in the door. Anne's asthma isn't aspirin-sensitive and she's taking NSAIDs to alleviate her discomfort. However, she sometimes has trouble pushing the pill out from the packet.

One afternoon, Anne suffers a severe asthma attack. After a night in hospital, she and the asthma nurse try to uncover why the attack occurred – Anne's asthma is usually well controlled. Anne admits that she's experienced problems actuating her MDI: she just can't seem to push hard enough. In addition, while her self-management plan suggests taking prednisolone tablets when her peak flow falls below 50 per cent of the predicted level, she cannot open the bottle's childproof cap. The asthma nurse switches to a DPI and the pharmacist provides both her asthma and arthritis medication in easy-to-open bottles.

Physical problems using inhalers

Some people with arthritis in their hands or difficulty holding certain inhalers find that devices called the Haleraid or Turboaid help.

- The Haleraid fits on to certain MDIs and allows you to apply pressure with the palm of your hand to activate the canister.
- The Turboaid fits on to the breath-actuated Turbohalers.

Ask your doctor, pharmacist or asthma nurse for further advice.

7

Coping with asthma: beyond drugs

Drugs are the mainstay of asthma management, preventing exacerbations, alleviating symptoms and enhancing quality of life. But regularly taking your preventer and using your reliever as required aren't the only steps you can take to improve control of your asthma. As this chapter illustrates, avoiding triggers, taking up vaccination, quitting smoking, losing weight, addressing psychological factors, improving your diet and using complementary therapies can all, combined with your drug treatment, help you cope with asthma.

Try to avoid the trigger

Obviously, you should do your best to avoid your particular asthma triggers. But you need to be realistic. Avoiding some triggers is easier said than done, and a single approach is unlikely to make much difference to symptoms triggered by some allergens, such as house dust mite. Moreover, some methods can be expensive, and studies have assessed relatively few of these in adults. Some of the recommendations below are based on studies on children, so if you try them it might be worth keeping a diary to see if your symptoms improve.

Pollen

The type of pollen in the air depends on the time of year and the weather; concentrations of grass pollen usually peak in June and July, for example, but the grass pollen season can, depending on the climate, run from May to August. In contrast, levels of birch pollen usually peak in April, while nettle tends to release pollen between June and September. If allergy tests reveal you are sensitive to a particular pollen, try to reduce your exposure during the times when levels are likely to be highest.

It's worth listening to, or visiting the webpage for, the weather forecast, which often warns when the pollen count is likely to be especially high. And on any given day, levels are likely to be higher at certain times. Grass pollen counts tend to peak in the morning and late afternoon of warm, dry days with a gentle wind, for example. You could consider staying indoors as far as possible, particularly in the early evening, when the weather forecast announces the pollen count is likely to be high.

Apart from keeping an eye on the weather, the following suggestions may reduce the risk that pollen will trigger an asthma attack (and hay fever if you suffer from both):

- Keep windows at home and in cars closed. You could ask your garage whether a new car has the option of special filters that reduce the amount of pollen that gets inside. In some cases, you may be able to fit the filters retrospectively.
- Pollen is sticky, so wash your hair regularly and change your clothes after being outside. A moustache can hold pollen right under your nose – make sure you shampoo any facial hair. Wash or wipe any pets that have been outside, especially if they've been in long grass or a wood.
- Get someone else to cut the grass. Obviously, this is especially important if you're allergic to grass pollen.
- Don't camp or picnic inland: try to holiday by the sea. Pollen counts tend to be lower on the coast than inland.
- Stock your home and garden with plants that produce relatively low levels of pollen, such as hibiscus, periwinkles, azaleas and roses. (Many people who think they're allergic to roses are actually sensitive to grass pollen.)

House dust mite

Even a powerful vacuum cleaner won't eradicate house dust mites: millions still call the most vigorously cleaned house their home. Indeed, some studies suggest that dry vacuum cleaners remove only between 5 and 30 per cent of the dust in a carpet. Other studies suggest that thorough vacuum cleaning may remove 70 per cent of mites – it depends on the cleaner, the conditions (such as the type of carpet) and how thoroughly the person vacuums. Wet vacuum and steam cleaners may remove more dust and mites – up to 80 per cent in some studies. However effective your cleaner, mites still breed rapidly so numbers return to the previous levels within a week or so. Nevertheless, while it's difficult to keep the dust and levels of mite allergens from building up, regular vacuuming can still help.

You'll probably need to combine several approaches to make a marked difference to levels of house dust mite. For example, beds are often the most important site of mite exposure. After all, you probably spend around a third of your life asleep. Many people allergic to the house dust mite encase their mattress in a protective cover. However, the level of exposure to mite allergens also depends on whether other items of bedding are covered or washed regularly. So, to tackle house dust mites, try the following:

- Wash bed linen using a cycle above 60°C, which kills the mites. Colder water washes away the allergen, but does not kill the mite.
- Put soft toys in the freezer or, if they won't be damaged, wash them in hot water every 14 days.
- Use dust mite (or anti-allergy) covers on mattresses, duvets and pillows. The covers may not alleviate symptoms in everyone, but some people find they help.
- House dust mites like it hot. Turn the central heating down and open windows.
- Consider decorating with wooden flooring and blinds rather than carpets and thick curtains. Wooden floors and blinds are easier to wash. If you really want a carpet, buy one with a very short pile.
- When you buy new furniture, consider leather or other nonporous surfaces, which makes cleaning easier.
- Avoid clutter, which can become dusty and is often difficult to clean. Keep books and knick-knacks in a box rather than on shelves, and store your belongings in cupboards.
- Vacuum cleaning can shift allergen from the floor to the air. Using double walled bags and cleaners fitted with HEPA or electrostatic filters may reduce the amount of dust that vacuuming creates. If possible, ask someone else to vacuum. Otherwise, wear a mask and, whoever vacuums, try not to re-enter a room for at least three hours after dusting or vacuuming to allow airborne dust to resettle.
- Ionizers increase the electrical charge on airborne dust particles, which clump together and fall to the ground, thus reducing the amount you inhale. It sounds logical. But there's no conclusive, scientific proof that ionizers improve asthma symptoms. Nonetheless, some people feel they help. (I used one on my desk for a while and it seemed to help. But that's no guarantee it'll work for you.)
- Some people find their symptoms improve after using miticides, which kill the mites. But follow the instructions carefully: some miticides can cause skin irritation.
- Remove sheepskins, which seem to harbour particularly large mite populations.
- The American College of Allergy, Asthma and Immunology suggests maintaining humidity below 55 per cent – so don't use a humidifier or a vaporizer.

Pet dander

Understandably, many people with asthma don't want to rehome their pets – they're part of the family. You will want to be certain that the animals cause your symptoms before deciding to find them a new home. (Ask for an allergy test, which may rule out the pets as causes.) You could also try the following to reduce levels of dander:

- Wash bed linen at about 60°C.
- Wash soft toys at least once a fortnight,
- Keep pets off beds and other soft furnishings.
- Avoid feather pillows. Many people allergic to animal dander cross-react to feathers.
- Ask someone who is not allergic to wash and comb your pet. If you must groom the pet, wear a mask and gloves.

People allergic to dander and other animals should remember that pet owners and others who work with animals may inadvertently transport dander on their clothing.

Fungi

As we saw in Chapter 2, fungi inside and outside the house can trigger asthma in sensitive people. You can reduce your exposure to indoor fungi in several ways:

- Regularly wipe any visible mould from bathrooms and windows with cleaners containing an antifungal or a 5 per cent bleach solution. (Wear a mask and non-latex gloves.) Make sure you clean shower curtains, tiles, shower stall, tub and toilet tank. Don't carpet the bathroom.
- Wash down walls with an antifungal before decorating. Use paints that contain an antifungal.
- Keep rooms dry and well ventilated. You could use a dehumidifier to keep the humidity below 50 per cent. Use the fan or open the window to reduce mould while bathing or cooking. Dry all clothing immediately after washing.
- High-efficiency particulate air filtration and air conditioning may reduce the amount of airborne antigen and alleviate asthma symptoms in individuals with fungal allergies.
- Convection heaters reduce the viability of mould spores and inhibit the spread of mildew.
- Bark often contains high levels of mould. If you use a fireplace or wood-burning stove, don't store any firewood inside (or, if there is no alternative, only a day's supply).

- Avoid foam rubber pillows and mattresses, which may be more likely to attract mould than other types of bedding.
- Wardrobes are often damp and dark and attract mould. Make sure you dry shoes and boots thoroughly before storing. You could use a chemical moisture-remover inside wardrobes.
- Empty the waste bin frequently. Keep the bins clean to prevent mould.
- Empty the drip pan under your refrigerator regularly. The combination of food particles and standing water is an ideal breeding ground for mould.

Vaccination

Flu

In the spring of 2009, Edgar Hernandez – a 5-year-old from La Gloria, a rural town some 155 miles east of Mexico City – suffered a fever and headache so intense that his eyes hurt. Edgar was the earliest confirmed case of the strain of 'swine flu' called H1N1/2009. He survived, but over the next 18 months around 18,500 people worldwide died from the infection and hundreds of thousands suffered severe symptoms, according to *The Lancet*.

Although experts had long predicted a flu pandemic, most expected a bird-flu strain arising in South Asia to sweep the world – but a pig farm close to La Gloria is probably ground zero for H1N1/2009. And some virologists foresaw a catastrophe, warning that a repeat of the 1918 Spanish flu pandemic could claim between 180 million and 360 million lives. Thankfully, H1N1/2009 killed fewer people than many seasonal outbreaks: 474 people died during the 2009–10 pandemic in the UK, while according to government figures 1,965 people died from flu in the 2004–5 winter season, 10,351 in 2008–9 season and 21,497 in 1999–2000.

But the fears and the death rates even in non-epidemic years show that influenza isn't just a bad cold. Flu is potentially fatal, especially for people with chronic respiratory diseases (including severe asthma, COPD or bronchitis), heart conditions and certain other ailments. Older people are also more likely to suffer serious complications – such as bronchitis or pneumonia – if they contract flu. So it's important to get your flu jab.

However, government figures suggest that only around 70 per cent of patients over 65 years of age were immunized with the seasonal flu vaccine during 2009–10, and only around half of high-risk patients (including those with severe asthma) below 65 years of age. If you are in a vulnerable group, your GP surgery should offer you a flu jab. If you feel you should have the jab but aren't offered it, speak to your GP or practice nurse.

Pneumonia (pneumococcal vaccination)

Around 1 per cent of the UK population contract pneumonia annually, especially during the autumn and winter. During a bout of pneumonia, fluid accumulates in the inflamed alveoli and small airways. This makes breathing difficult and reduces the amount of oxygen that passes into the blood. Most people feel ill and are feverish and 'off their food' for a few days. However, in 2008, almost 29,000 people in the UK died from pneumonia. Although a plethora of pathogens potentially cause pneumonia, bacteria cause around half of all cases.

Doctors may advocate pneumococcal vaccine for people with asthma or for adults aged at least 65 years. *Streptococcus pneumoniae*, the agent that causes many cases of pneumonia, can also lead to blood poisoning (septicaemia) and meningitis. The vaccines used in the elderly and high-risk groups may reduce the risk of pneumonia and other serious pneumococcal diseases by between 50 and 70 per cent.

While vaccination makes sense, there is surprisingly little evidence that asthmatic adults benefit. Nevertheless, a study of asthmatic children by Sheikh and colleagues found that pneumococcal vaccination decreased the number of acute asthma exacerbations from ten to seven per child per year. We clearly need further studies. But as pneumonia is potentially so dangerous, it's worth discussing vaccination with your doctor or nurse.

Quit smoking

Smoking is rapidly becoming socially unacceptable – just look at the huddles of smokers outside offices, pubs and restaurants. During the 1940s, around 70 per cent of men and 40 per cent of women smoked. According to government statistics, the proportion of adults in England who smoke fell from 28 to 21 per cent between 1998 and 2008. Nevertheless, in England more than a fifth of adults – about 8.8 million people – still smoke. Around half of those who don't quit smoking will die prematurely from their addiction. Indeed, during 2008 more than 80,000 people died prematurely in England from smoking-related diseases. For example:

- Smokers are roughly twice as likely to die from cancer as non-smokers.
- Smoking causes around half of all cases of heart disease.

- Smoking increases the likelihood of suffering a stroke up to three-fold.
- Smoking underlies a fifth of deaths among middle-aged people.

As we've mentioned before, smoking (even second-hand) exacerbates asthma and makes the disease more difficult to control. For example, smoking seems to reduce the effectiveness of inhaled steroids.

On the other hand, quitting smoking reduces your likelihood of developing the main smoking-related diseases and helps prevent exacerbations. According to the Department of Health, a lifelong smoker loses, on average, around ten years of life. A person who stops smoking at 30 or 40 years of age gains, on average, ten or nine years of life respectively. Even a 60-year-old gains three years of life by quitting. So, it's never too late to quit.

If the benefits to your health are not enough to make you quit, think of the harm you're doing to the people around you. Second-hand smoke contains more than 4,000 chemicals, including over 50 carcinogens. This chemical cocktail increases the risk of asthma attacks and other serious diseases – including lung cancer, heart disease, childhood respiratory disease and sudden infant death syndrome – in people who inhale second-hand smoke. For example, the risks that a woman who has never smoked will develop lung cancer and heart disease are 24 and 30 per cent greater, respectively, if she lives with a smoker.

However, fewer than one in every 30 smokers manages to quit each year, and of these more than half relapse within a year. And you need to quit, not cut down. People who reduce cigarette consumption usually inhale more deeply to get the same amount of nicotine. Nevertheless, cutting back does seem to increase the likelihood that you'll eventually quit. In some studies, people who halved their cigarette consumption increased their chances of eventual cessation by 70 per cent compared with those who never cut back. In other words, reduction can take you a large step towards kicking the habit. But don't stop there.

You'll need to deal with nicotine's withdrawal symptoms, which can leave you irritable, restless and anxious as well as experiencing insomnia and craving a cigarette. In general, these withdrawal symptoms abate over two weeks or so. But nicotine replacement therapy (NRT) can make life a little easier. Government statistics suggest that nearly a fifth of smokers buy NRT to aid cessation. It's money well spent: NRT increases quit rates by between 50 and 100 per cent.

You can chose from various types of NRT. Patches reduce withdrawal symptoms but have a relatively slow onset of action while nicotine chewing gum, lozenges, inhalers and nasal spray act more quickly. Talk to your pharmacist or doctor to find the right combination for you. If you still find quitting tough even after trying NRT, doctors can prescribe other treatments. But there's no quick fix. You'll still need to be committed to quitting.

Tips to help you quit

Breaking tobacco's hold is tough. But, in addition to using NRT, a few simple hints may make life easier:

• Set a quit date, when you will stop completely. Plan ahead: keep a diary of problems and situations that tempt you to light up, such as meals, pubs or breaks at work. Many people associate tobacco with alcohol and coffee, for example.
• Try to find something to take your mind off smoking. If you find yourself smoking when you get home in the evening, try a new hobby or exercise. Most people find that the craving for a cigarette usually only lasts a couple of minutes. Some people find that just sucking a hard sweet helps take their mind off the craving.
• You may want to ask your family and friends for advice and support.
• Smoking is expensive. Keep a note of how much you save and spend at least some of it on something special for yourself.
• Some people find that they become more hungry when they lose weight, so try to avoid reaching for the chocolate. Have a healthy snack handy.

Coping with relapses

Nicotine is incredibly addictive, on some measures more addictive than heroin and cocaine. Not surprisingly, many people don't manage to quit first time – tobacco's grip is just too strong. But if you relapse, try not to become too dispirited. Regard it as a temporary setback rather than meaning you are permanently hooked. Set yourself another quit date and try again.

It's also worth trying to identify why you relapsed. Were you stressed out? If so, why? Did you met up with particular friends? Was smoking linked to a particular time, place or event? Once you know why you slipped you can develop strategies to stop the problem in the future.

Losing weight

According to government statistics, 24 per cent of men and 25 per cent of women in England are obese. Furthermore, 42 per cent of men and 32 per cent of women are overweight. Apart from increasing your risk of developing type 2 diabetes, heart disease and some cancers (including colon, kidney and breast), excess weight can exacerbate your asthma symptoms. And as we've already seen, obesity is a risk factor for severe asthma. Indeed, obese and overweight asthmatics typically show greater airway obstruction and are more likely to endure nocturnal symptoms than those who maintain a healthy weight.

On the other hand, losing weight alleviates symptoms and improves diurnal and day-to-day variations in peak flow, FEV_1 and airway resistance. In part, these improvements result from the reductions in the amount of fat within or pressing down on the airways. Fat can narrow and change the airway's shape from a circle to a less efficient oval. Abdominal fat may also prevent the diaphragm from descending as far as in people of a healthy weight. Last but not least, obese people tend to have smaller lung volumes than those of healthy weight.

In part, the link between excess weight and asthma arises because fat isn't just inert blubber – it's a chemical factory. Cells that make up fat (adipocytes) pump out several chemical messengers that increase inflammation in the lungs and other parts of the body. So, as Mancuso points out, excessive fat deposits increase susceptibility to pulmonary infections and exacerbate the airway inflammation associated with environmental triggers.

Losing any excess weight is not easy: after all, millions of years of evolution drive us to consume food in times of feast to help us survive during times of famine. (Today, of course, few people in the Western world experience famine. But the drive to eat hasn't changed so we pile on the pounds.) And you can't stop eating as you can quit smoking. However, the following six tips may help:

- Try to take 30 to 60 minutes of aerobic exercise each day. That doesn't necessarily mean training for a marathon: brisk walking, jogging, taking an aerobics class or using a machine like a stationary bike or treadmill will all help you lose weight. You don't even need to do it in one go. You can break the exercise down into chunks of 10 or 15 minutes.
- Keep a food diary and record everything you eat and drink for a couple of weeks. It's often easy to see where you inadvertently pile on the extra calories: the odd biscuit here, the extra glass of wine or full-fat latte there. It all adds up. You could use one of the online tools that estimate your calorie intake and track weight loss over time (see Useful addresses).
- Be realistic: don't try to lose too much weight too quickly. Few people keep the weight off if they crash diet. Steadily losing around a pound or two a week reduces your chance of putting it back on again.

- Be specific. Don't say that you want to lose weight: rather, resolve to lose two stone. (Several internet sites allow you to estimate your body mass index and ideal weight, which helps you set yourself a target, such as <http://www.nhs.uk/Tools/Pages/Healthyweightcalculator. aspx>. Alternately, ask your doctor, practice nurse or pharmacist to calculate your body mass index for you.)
- Set yourself small attainable goals, such as switching from full fat to skimmed milk, walking 15 minutes during your lunch break each day, going to the gym three times a week, and only indulging in chocolate on Fridays.
- Don't let a slip-up derail your diet. Try to identify why you indulged – what were the triggers? A particular occasion? Stress? Once you know why you slipped you can develop strategies to stop the problem in the future.

If all this fails, try talking to your GP. A growing number of medicines may help kick-start your weight loss. None of these tips is a magic cure for being overweight and you'll still need to change your lifestyle. However, you may find that they help put you on the right course towards weight loss.

Psychological factors

Living with asthma – or any chronic disease – can cause considerable stress and have a marked impact on your family, social and work life. And you live with a lingering fear that you'll suffer a severe, perhaps life-threatening, exacerbation. So, not surprisingly, suffering from asthma can cause or exacerbate anxiety, depression and other psychiatric ailments. In turn, suffering from some psychiatric conditions can make your asthma worse.

For example, Schmitz and colleagues found that in the two weeks preceding their study, 17 per cent of those with asthma and low levels of psychological distress had spent time in bed or reduced normal activities for all or most of the day because of asthma. This compared with 35 per cent of asthmatics with moderate psychological distress and 69 per cent of those enduring high levels of psychological distress.

Indeed, some psychiatric problems may trigger asthma, perhaps by unmasking a pre-existing disease. Loerbroks and colleagues found that patients that scored highly on questionnaires measuring neuroticism (a personality trait linked to stress) were around three times more likely to develop asthma than those with low scores on this trait. Divorce or the end of a 'life partnership' approximately doubled the likelihood of developing asthma.

Depression

Depression and anxiety also seem to worsen asthma. Depression is more than being 'a bit down': it's a profound feeling of debilitating mental and physical lethargy, a pervasive sense of worthlessness and intense, deep, unshakable sadness. If you've never experienced true depression, it's difficult to appreciate just how devastating the condition can be. Ng and co-researchers found that among patients aged 60 years and above, asthma roughly doubled the likelihood of suffering from depression compared with people without asthma and other chronic illnesses.

Not surprisingly, depression compromises our ability to solve problems. In many cases, the strategies a depressed person develops to cope with asthma make matters worse. For example, if you are depressed this can induce a profound lethargy that saps your will and undermines your motivation to follow your doctor's or nurse's advice on when to use your medications for asthma and other diseases. In other cases, you may deny that you suffer from asthma – depression shunts the condition to the back of your mind.

Anxiety

Anxiety is more than feeling a little wound up, worried or stressed out. It's a feeling of intense, sometimes debilitating, fear – even abject terror. Asthma, especially if severe or poorly controlled, can cause considerable anxiety. After all, asthma attacks are often frightening and the next attack could be the one that proves fatal. Not surprisingly, people with asthma are especially likely to develop anxiety disorders, including:

- generalized anxiety – anxiety all the time;
- panic disorder – unpredictable, intense anxiety attacks (according to the Royal College of Psychiatrists, around a quarter of people who go to an A&E department suffering from chest pain have suffered a panic attack rather than a heart attack);
- social phobia – intense anxiety when you are with other people.

To make matters worse, anxiety stimulates the adrenal glands (on top of your kidneys) to pour adrenaline into your bloodstream, causing your breathing to become faster to take in more oxygen. Obviously, changes to respiration worry asthmatics. The adrenaline rush also heightens alertness and the senses, increasing awareness of the changes. It's easy to become trapped in a self-perpetuating cycle of anxiety and asthma.

Once again, anxiety can compromise your ability to take rational decisions about your asthma. For example, you need to be alert for signs of worsening asthma and severe attacks. But anxiety can lead to you becoming over-cautious, so you may needlessly use medication, attend A&E or miss work. And if you are anxious about side effects, you may not use your inhaler as needed.

Stress and the immune system

Stress can affect the immune system – which makes biological sense. Essentially, the biological changes associated with stress evolved to protect us from potential physical threats by allowing us to fight back or run away, so the increased immune activity allows stress to prepare us to tackle an infection.

Unfortunately, excessive stress (especially if protracted) may undermine your immune defences. For example, natural killer cells, a type of white blood cell, attack and destroy infected or cancerous cells. One study of students found that the activity of the natural killer cells declined around the time of their examinations. Indeed, several studies suggest that excessive stress reduces the effectiveness of some types of white blood cell and increases the risk of infection. One study infected students experimentally with influenza virus. Stressed-out students suffered worse symptoms and produced more mucus than their less worried counterparts. These changes would be bad news for people with asthma.

Other studies confirm that stress affects the immune system. For example, your immune system needs to mount an adequate response (such as pumping out sufficiently high levels of protective antibodies) after a vaccination to reduce your chances of contracting the infection. However, in one study, carers looking after a husband or wife with dementia found that levels of a cytokine (chemical mediator) that increases the activity of the immune system rose more quickly and persisted for longer after a vaccination than in less chronically stressed adults. In another study, carers generated lower levels of protective antibodies following a flu jab. Overall, Byrne-Davis and Vedhara comment, chronic stress can prematurely age the immune response.

Getting help

It's important to get help for depression, anxiety and any other psychiatric conditions. If symptoms have a marked impact on your daily life, the doctor may suggest anti-depressants or drugs to alleviate anxiety. Don't dismiss these out of hand. As mentioned above, it's often difficult to plan the most appropriate strategy for your asthma or your life when you're carrying the burden of depression or anxiety. While drugs can ease the symptoms, they don't cure the problem. Nevertheless, psychiatric medicines may offer you a 'window of opportunity' to improve your asthma control and deal with any other life issues you currently face.

You could, for example, learn more about asthma and discuss steps you can take to improve your control with your doctor or asthma nurse. A change in your asthma medication may improve your symptoms and, in turn, reduce your anxiety or depression. You might want to discuss ways to improve your adherence with your treatment or tackle some of the triggers around your home. Putting yourself in control of your problems is one of the best ways to beat anxiety and depression. On the other hand, feeling that your problems control you is one of the most common causes of anxiety, depression and stress.

Nevertheless, some people need additional help. Your GP may be able to recommend a local counsellor. Alternatively, you could contact the British Association for Counselling and Psychotherapy or see if your doctor can refer you on the NHS. 'Talking therapies', such as cognitive behavioural therapy (CBT), help you identify the feelings, thoughts and behaviours that you associate with asthma. CBT will then help you question and test the feelings, thoughts, behaviours and beliefs to discover those that are unhelpful and unrealistic. In other words, CBT helps you face issues you have been avoiding and try out new ways of behaving and reacting. Furthermore, many complementary therapies (see below) help you relax, which bolsters your defences against stress.

Diet

You are what you eat, but studies examining the effect of diet on asthma show mixed results. For example, some studies, but not all, suggest that high levels of salt in the diet increase airway responsiveness.

Furthermore, Inuits seem to be less vulnerable to several diseases, including diabetes, heart disease and asthma, than people in Western countries, despite living on a diet that consists almost entirely of meat and living in a very cold environment. But their diets are high in fish and animals that eat fish (such as seals). Some fish oils (n-3, also called omega-3, fatty acids) appear to be anti-inflammatory, which may be why Inuits are at lower risk. Certainly, some studies suggest that diets high in oily fish (such as mackerel, fresh tuna and fresh salmon) seem to protect against asthma. Other studies have found that, in smokers, consumption of fish and n-3 fatty acids reduced the risk of emphysema, chronic bronchitis and low spirometry values. But not all studies have found a benefit.

While these results are mixed, reducing salt consumption also protects against raised blood pressure, while diets high in oily fish seem to protect against several other conditions, including heart disease. It's less clear whether supplements offer any benefit over increasing fatty fish consumption, although they may be an alternative for people who really don't like fatty fish. You could increase your consumption of fatty fish and see if your symptoms improve.

Furthermore, as mentioned in Chapter 2, some additives and preservatives (e.g. tartrazine) and certain foods (notably milk, egg and wheat) may precipitate asthma in sensitive people. However, you shouldn't start cutting milk, egg and other basic foods from your diet without advice from a dietician. If you feel that foods exacerbate your symptoms, you should discuss your concerns with your doctor or asthma nurse.

Complementary treatments

Complementary medicines are increasingly popular. A postal survey of 1,308 asthma patients in England performed by Shaw and collaborators during 2005–6 found that 15 per cent had used complementary therapies. Around a fifth (18 per cent) used the therapy to help their asthma, such as opening their airways. Other common reasons included a belief that the therapy was natural or safe (12 per cent), a recommendation by a family member or friend (12 per cent), and to aid relaxation and calm breathing (8 per cent).

Homeopathy emerged as the most popular complementary treatment among asthmatics (used by 68 per cent), followed by herbal treatments (63 per cent), relaxation (56 per cent), acupuncture (46 per cent) and the Buteyko breathing method (41 per cent). Obviously, some people tried more than one therapy.

Many of the people with asthma felt they benefited from the complementary treatment. Shaw and colleagues found that more than half said that the therapy always (23 per cent) or usually (33 per cent) helped their asthma. A further 28 per cent said that the complementary treatment sometimes helped. Fewer asthma symptoms (reported by 44 per cent) and helping to calm breathing and reduce panic (37 per cent) were the most common benefits.

Nevertheless, many conventional doctors and nurses remain cynical, partly because few complementary therapies undergo the same rigorous scrutiny as modern medicines. But clinical studies are expensive and pharmaceutical companies fund most trials, so this lack of studies isn't that surprising. It's worth remembering that no evidence of effectiveness isn't necessarily the same as evidence of no effect.

Cynics add that the placebo effect accounts for most of the benefits produced by complementary medicines. In other words, if you think that treatment will work, you'll probably feel better. (We've already seen that the immune system and nervous system are intimately linked.) And the symptoms and severity of asthma wax and wane, so symptoms may improve without treatment. Even without treatment, many mild or moderate exacerbations will fade to your average daily symptoms. (Doctors call this 'regression to the mean' – the mean is the average.)

That's undoubtedly true. However, the placebo effect and the natural resolution also contribute to conventional medicines' benefits. Because of this, many studies of conventional drugs compare the treatment to a placebo – a tablet or inhaler that looks the same as the medicine but doesn't contain any active ingredient. In the best-designed studies, neither the patient nor the doctor knows whether the treatment is active or a placebo. (The technical term is a 'double-blind' study.) Kemeny and colleagues examined the placebo response in 55 patients with mild intermittent and persistent asthma and stable airway hyper-reactivity. The placebo (inactive) bronchodilator reduced bronchial hyper-reactivity: the average concentration of methacholine needed to reduce FEV_1 by 20 per cent nearly doubled. Asthmatic symptoms 'responded' to the placebo in 18 per cent of patients.

Furthermore, cynics may point out that few studies show that complementary therapies improve lung function in people with asthma. However, improvements in measures of asthma control – such as limitation of activity, shortness of breath and wheezing – are not necessarily linked to changes in lung function. (A treatment may reduce over-inflation of lungs, for example.) This means that a complementary therapy may still improve symptoms and enhance quality of life, even if peak flow doesn't change markedly.

And some complementary therapies make sense biologically. If a technique improves breathing, it's logical that it might improve asthma. Even treatments that – from the perspective of conventional medicine – seem to lack any rational scientific basis may help. Reflexology, for example, can help you relax, and this, in turn, will help alleviate stress-related symptoms and improve your quality of life even without, according to conventional medicine, any direct impact on the causes of asthma.

Don't underestimate relaxation's benefits! Hypnosis and other relaxation therapies benefited asthma in two of five well-designed trials. Muscle relaxation could conceivably improve lung function in patients with asthma. So, if you want to try a complementary therapy, learn as much as you can about the treatment, see a reputable therapist and keep a diary of symptoms to see if there is any improvement. Bear in mind that stress may make your asthma worse.

Do regard these as *complementary* – not alternative – medicines. Don't stop taking your conventional medicines, and make sure your asthma nurse or doctor knows – even if he or she is cynical. A common misconception suggests that because complementary therapies are natural they are therefore safe. However, many complementary therapies can also cause side effects: some herbs, for example, can be highly toxic and interact with other drugs you're taking. You should always talk to your doctor or asthma nurse before trying a complementary treatment.

If you feel that the therapy improves your symptoms and you feel ready to step down your conventional treatment, speak to your doctor or asthma nurse before cutting back. (You should be regularly reviewed in any case and the treatment reduced to the minimum that controls symptoms; see Chapter 6.) In general, provided there's no medical reason why you shouldn't and if you find it improves your quality of life, it may be worth trying a complementary treatment – even if it 'just' helps you relax.

Acupuncture

Many people with asthma report that acupuncture alleviates their symptoms, although the evidence from clinical trials is mixed. For example, Choi and colleagues reported that 12 sessions of acupuncture added to conventional treatment over four weeks did not improve average morning peak flow or FEV_1 in asthmatic adults. However, quality of life and Transition Dyspnoea Index – a questionnaire measuring breathlessness related to activities of daily living – both improved. While the extent of acupuncture's benefits remains a moot point, some people find this ancient technique alleviates their symptoms and improves their quality of life.

Alexander therapy

Alexander therapy aims to re-educate the body, correct bad posture, bring the body into 'natural alignment' and aid relaxation. In some ways, it makes sense that Alexander therapy may benefit asthma. As we saw in Chapter 1, the chest needs to stretch optimally during inhalation and exhalation. Bad posture can hinder the chest's movement and compress the airways, so opening the airways by improving bad posture seems logical.

Many actors, musicians and singers find that the Alexander technique enhances their ability to project their voice and improves stamina. Some asthma patients find that the Alexander technique improves their symptoms and reduces their need for medicine. Indeed, one small study suggested that the Alexander technique improved lung function; peak flow improved by 9 per cent, for example. However, after examining the scientific studies Dennis concluded that there is too little scientific evidence to suggest the Alexander technique alleviates asthma, although some people undoubtedly feel it helps.

Breathing techniques

Before modern drugs, many patients and physicians relied on breathing exercises to control asthma symptoms. However, despite the advent of modern drugs many asthma patients still show poor breathing techniques that could, in some cases, make their symptoms worse. For instance, people with asthma may breathe through their mouth only, or may not use their chest muscles correctly. Other people with asthma breathe too rapidly (hyperventilation).

Dysfunctional breathing can exacerbate asthma and, in some cases, even trigger attacks. So, there now seems little doubt that learning to breathe correctly can improve asthma. And there's been a resurgence of interest in recent years, partly in the wake of patients reporting impressive results with yogic breathing and the Buteyko method. In addition to any direct effect on asthma symptoms, several breathing techniques, such as those derived from yoga or Buddhist meditation, can help you relax.

Against this background, doctors at Papworth Hospital near Cambridge developed a sequence of breathing and relaxation exercises for asthma during the 1960s. When you're stressed or anxious you probably take rapid, shallow breaths using, predominately, the muscles at the top of your chest. The Papworth technique counters this 'over-breathing' by encouraging more relaxed breathing using the abdomen and diaphragm. Essentially, patients drop their shoulders, relax their abdomens and breathe deeply and calmly. Holloway and West reported that six months after people had spent five sessions learning the technique, the severity of asthma symptoms had declined by around a third; a year later, symptom severity had still declined by a quarter. Although most objective measures of lung function showed no change, the technique also alleviated anxiety and depression.

Yoga and Buteyko breathing techniques aim to control hyperventilation by reducing respiration rate. Doctors who reviewed the studies assessing these techniques concluded that breathing exercises do not change lung function. However, one study found that a yogic breath-control exercise called pranayama slightly reduces airway responsiveness to histamine (see challenge tests, p. 64). Furthermore, several trials suggest that while Buteyko does not enhance lung function, symptoms improve and bronchodilator use declines.

In another study, a physiotherapist taught breathing exercises to people with poorly controlled mild to moderate asthma over three sessions. Thomas and colleagues commented that, six months after learning the breathing exercises, patients reported improved asthma-related quality of life compared to a group who received education about the disease from a nurse: in these two groups, 91 per cent and 64 per cent respectively showed a 'clinically important' improvement in asthma-related quality of life. (Of course, the study also underscores the benefit of education in asthma.) Patients who had learnt the breathing exercises reported less anxiety and depression, although neither airway inflammation nor hyper-responsiveness had changed.

Herbal medicine

Some herbal remedies undoubtedly alleviate asthma. For example, one review reported that nine out of 17 trials examining herbal treatments reported some improvement in lung function. However, determining which herbs work can be difficult: one Chinese herb decoction (*Ding Chuan Tang*), which improved airway hyper-responsiveness in children with stable asthma, contains nine components, so more than one plant may be responsible for the benefits and each plant may contain thousands of potentially active ingredients.

Indeed, numerous herbs used in traditional medicines worldwide are anti-inflammatory, act as bronchodilators or help you deal with stress and anxiety. (While it doesn't mean that it will work for you, I've found herbal remedies invaluable for asthma and other conditions over the years.) However, some herbs can interfere with other drugs or cause side effects. As mentioned in Chapter 2, some herbs contain salicylates and may therefore trigger symptoms in people with aspirin-sensitive asthma. So, if you want to try herbal treatments, ensure that you contact a registered medical herbalist and inform your GP, nurse, pharmacist and other healthcare professionals.

Homeopathy

Few alternative treatments provoke as much controversy as homeopathy. Based on the idea that like treats like, homeopathy uses a very dilute preparation of a chemical that produces the same symptoms as the disease, e.g. grass or ragweed for people allergic to those plants. According to conventional medicine these dilutions are simply too low to have any biological effect, so any benefit is down to the placebo effect and natural resolution.

Yet the idea that homeopathy works remains remarkably persistent. Quite apart from thousands of anecdotal stories, a review found that two of three methodologically sound randomized controlled trials reported some positive effects. However, these studies did not make the homeopathic treatment specific to each individual, which practitioners say is essential to gain the full benefit. And many doctors criticize the rigour of the limited scientific evidence that supports homeopathy.

On the other hand, if homeopathy doesn't have a biological action it won't do you any harm provided you take your conventional medicines. If you want to try homeopathy, you need to balance the lack of a scientific basis and the dearth, in many doctors' view, of rigorous studies against the anecdotal reports. If you decide to proceed, keep a diary to see if your symptoms improve and for how long. (Indeed, this is a good idea for any complementary medicine.) This can then help you decide whether it's worth the money.

A final word

Over the course of this book, we've seen that asthma is common: doctors currently treat around 4.3 million adults for asthma in the UK alone. Adults are also more likely to die from asthma than children. Tragically, better care could prevent up to 90 per cent of deaths and 75 per cent of admissions to hospital due to asthma, as well as enhancing quality of life, helping you perform the normal activities of daily life everyone else seems to take for granted and reducing the time you take sick from work. So, you need to get your asthma under control.

Nevertheless, asthma in adults often doesn't receive the attention it deserves. While children and adults share several risk factors and the broad approaches to treatment are similar, there are some important differences. To take one obvious example, work-related factors cause up to a quarter of asthma cases among adults and contribute to approximately 15 per cent of severe exacerbations. However, combining treatments, avoiding triggers and considering other interventions should help you cope with asthma.

Useful addresses

Allergy UK
Planwell House
LEFA Business Park
Edgington Way
Sidcup
Kent DA14 5BH
Tel.: 01322 619898 (helpline)
Website: www.allergyuk.org

Asthma UK
Summit House
70 Wilson Street
London EC2A 2DB
Tel.: 0800 121 62 44 (adviceline);
0800 121 62 55 (general)
Website: www.asthma.org.uk

Asthma UK Cymru
Third Floor, Eastgate House
34–43 Newport Road
Cardiff CF24 0AB
Tel.: 02920 435 400

Asthma UK Northern Ireland
Ground Floor, Unit 2
College House
City Link Business Park
Durham Street
Belfast BT12 4HQ
Tel.: 0800 151 3035

Asthma UK Scotland
4 Queen Street
Edinburgh EH2 1JE
Tel.: 0131 226 2544

British Acupuncture Council
63 Jeddo Road
London W12 9HQ
Tel.: 020 8735 0400
Website: www.acupuncture.org.uk

British Association for Counselling and Psychotherapy
BACP House
15 St John's Business Park
Lutterworth
Leicestershire LE17 4HB
Tel.:01455 883300
Website: www.bacp.co.uk

British Lung Foundation
73–75 Goswell Road
London EC1V 7ER
Tel.: 020 7688 5555; helpline: 08458 50 50 20
Website: www.lunguk.org

Lung and Asthma Information Agency
Website: www.laia.ac.uk
An academic unit in the Department of Community Health Sciences
at St George's Hospital Medical School, University of London. Statistics
and factsheets on various respiratory conditions and diseases may be
freely downloaded.

National Health Service (for advice on stopping smoking)
NHS Smoking Helpline: 0800 022 4 332
Website: http://smokefree.nhs.uk

National Institute of Medical Herbalists
Elm House
54 Mary Arches Street
Exeter EX4 3BA
Tel. 01392 426022
Website: www.nimh.org.uk

Royal College of Psychiatrists
17 Belgrave Square
London SW1X 8PG
Tel.: 020 7235 2351
Website: www.rcpsych.ac.uk/default.aspx
Mental health information for patients:
www.rcpsych.ac.uk/mentalhealthinfoforall.aspx

Society of Homeopaths
11 Brookfield, Duncan Close
Moulton Park
Northampton NN3 6WL
Tel.: 0845 450 6611 or, if calling from outside the UK: 01604 817890
Website: www.homeopathy-soh.org

Society of Teachers of the Alexander Technique
First Floor, Linton House
39–51 Highgate Road
London NW5 1RS
Tel. 020 7482 5135
Website: www.stat.org.uk
If searching for a teacher, visit <www.statsearch.co.uk>

Other useful websites

American Academy of Allergy, Asthma and Immunology:
www.aaaai.org

Asthma Australia: www.asthmaaustralia.org

Asthma Society of Canada: www.asthma.ca

British Guideline on the Management of Asthma:
www.sign.ac.uk/guidelines/fulltext/101/index.html.

Cochrane reviews: www.thecochranelibrary.com
Although primarily aimed at healthcare professionals, each guideline
includes a summary for the general public.

European Respiratory Society: www.ersnet.org

Global Initiative for Asthma (GINA): www.ginasthma.com

Occupational Asthma (list of causes):
www.asthme.csst.qc.ca/document/Info_Gen/AgenProf/Bernstein/Bern-
steinAng.htm

References

A book such as this stands on the shoulders of research performed by clinicians and scientists worldwide. Unfortunately, it is impossible to include every paper and website that I consulted to write this book – and I apologize for any oversights. In addition to the reviews and books mentioned in the 'Further reading' section, the following studies illustrate particular points in each chapter and are referred to by name. You can access summaries, and in some cases the full paper, by entering the details here: < http://www.ncbi.nlm.nih.gov/pubmed>.

Introduction

Dean, B.B. *et al.*, 'The impact of uncontrolled asthma on absenteeism and health-related quality of life', *Journal of Asthma* 46 (2009): 861–6.

Partridge, M.R. *et al.*, 'Attitudes and actions of asthma patients on regular maintenance therapy: the INSPIRE study', *BMC Pulmonary Medicine* 6 (2006): 13.

Chapter 1

Anon, 'Bodily breeding', *New Scientist*, 30 September 2000, p. 97.

Elias, J.A., 'Airway remodeling in asthma', *American Journal of Respiratory and Critical Care Medicine* 161 (2000): S168–71.

Loerbroks, A. *et al.*, 'Neuroticism, extraversion, stressful life events and asthma: a cohort study of middle-aged adults', *Allergy* 64 (2009): 1444–50.

Moffat, M.A. *et al.*, 'Large-scale, consortium-based genomewide association study of asthma', *New England Journal of Medicine* 363 (2010): 1211–21.

Virchow, J.C., 'Intrinsic asthma', in W.W. Busse and S.T. Holgate (eds) *Asthma and Rhinitis*, Wiley-Blackwell, Oxford, second edn 2008.

Chapter 2

Adcock, I.M. and Barnes, P.J., 'Molecular mechanisms of corticosteroid resistance', *Chest* 134 (2008): 394–401.

Dharmage, S.C. *et al.*, 'Do childhood respiratory infections continue to influence adult respiratory morbidity?' *European Respiratory Journal* 33 (2009): 237–44.

Kuna, P. *et al.*, 'Severe asthma attacks after sexual intercourse', *American Journal of Respiratory and Critical Care Medicine* 170 (2004): 344–5.

Ségala, C. *et al.*, 'Asthma in adults: comparison of adult-onset asthma with childhood-onset asthma relapsing in adulthood', *Allergy* 55 (2000): 634–40.

Sinha, T. and David, A.K., 'Recognition and management of exercise-induced bronchospasm', *American Family Physician* 67 (2003): 675, 769–74.

Chapter 3

Bell, M.L., Davis, D.L. and Fletcher, T., 'A retrospective assessment of mortality from the London smog episode of 1952: the role of influenza and pollution', *Environmental Health Perspectives* 112 (2004): 6–8.

Bozek, A. and Jarzab, J., 'Adherence to asthma therapy in elderly patients', *Journal of Asthma* 47 (2010): 162–5.

Calhoun, W.J., 'Nocturnal asthma', *Chest* 123 (2003) 399S–405S.

Clatworthy, J., Price, D., Ryan, D. *et al.*, 'The value of self-report assessment of adherence, rhinitis and smoking in relation to asthma control', *Primary Care Respiratory Journal* 18 (2009): 300–5.

Conn, H.O. and Poynard, T., 'Corticosteroids and peptic ulcer: meta-analysis of adverse events during steroid therapy', *Journal of Internal Medicine* 236 (1994): 619–32.

D'Amato, G., Liccardi, G. and Frenguelli, G., 'Thunderstorm-asthma and pollen allergy', *Allergy* 62 (2007): 11–6.

Dean, N.L., 'Perimenstrual asthma exacerbations and positioning of leukotriene-modifying agents in asthma management guidelines', *Chest* 120 (2001): 2116–17.

Dratva, J., Schindler, C., Curjuric, I. *et al.*, 'Perimenstrual increase in bronchial hyperreactivity in premenopausal women: results from the population-based SAPALDIA 2 cohort', *Journal of Allergy and Clinical Immunology* 125 (2010): 823–9.

Fairs, A., Agbetile, J., Hargadon, B. *et al.*, 'IgE sensitization to *Aspergillus fumigatus* is associated with reduced lung function in asthma', *American Journal of Respiratory and Critical Care Medicine* 182 (2010): 1362–8.

Gibson, P.G., Henry, R. and Coughlan, J.J.L., 'Gastro-oesophageal reflux treatment for asthma in adults and children', *Cochrane Database of Systematic Reviews* (2003) CD001496.

Murphy, V.E. and Gibson, P.G., 'Premenstrual asthma: prevalence, cycle-to-cycle variability and relationship to oral contraceptive use and menstrual symptoms', *Journal of Asthma* 45 (2008): 696–704.

Murray, J.K., Browne, W.J., Roberts, M.A. *et al.*, 'Number and ownership profiles of cats and dogs in the UK', *Veterinary Record* 166 (2010): 163–8.

Öberg, M., Jaakkola, M.S., Woodward, A. *et al.*, 'Worldwide burden of disease from exposure to second-hand smoke: a retrospective analysis of data from 192 countries', *The Lancet* 377 (2011): 139–46.

Pereira-Vega, A., Sánchez, J.L., Gil, F.L. *et al.*, 'Premenstrual asthma and symptoms related to premenstrual syndrome', *Journal of Asthma* 47 (2010): 835–40.

Rachiotis, G., Savani, R., Brant, A. *et al.*, 'Outcome of occupational asthma after cessation of exposure: a systematic review', *Thorax* 62 (2007): 147–52.

Romieu, I., Fabre, A., Fournier, A. *et al*, 'Postmenopausal hormone therapy and asthma onset in the E3N cohort', *Thorax* 65 (2010): 292–7.

Ségala, C. *et al.*, 'Asthma in adults: comparison of adult-onset asthma with childhood-onset asthma relapsing in adulthood', *Allergy* 55 (2000): 634–40.

Ye, W., Chow, W.H., Lagergren, J. *et al.*, 'Risk of adenocarcinomas of the oesophagus and gastric cardia in patients hospitalized for asthma', *British Journal of Cancer* 85 (2001): 1317–21.

Chapter 4

The following is especially useful: P. Cullinan and A.J. Taylor, 'Occupational asthma', in A.B. Kay, A.P. Kaplan, J. Bousquet and P.G. Holt (eds) *Allergy and Allergic Diseases*, Wiley, New York, second edn 2009.

Aldrich, T.K., Gustave, J., Hall, C.B. *et al.*, 'Lung function in rescue workers at the World Trade Center after seven years', *New England Journal of Medicine* 362 (2010): 1263–72.

Ayres, J.G., Boyd, R., Cowie, H. *et al.*, 'Costs of occupational asthma in the UK', *Thorax* (2011) 66: 128–33.

Campbell, C.P. and Yates, D.H., 'Lupin allergy: a hidden killer at home, a menace at work; occupational disease due to lupin allergy', *Clinical and Experimental Allergy* 40 (2010): 1467–72.

Campo, P., Aranda, A., Rondon, C. *et al.*, 'Work-related sensitization and respiratory symptoms in carpentry apprentices exposed to wood dust and diisocyanates', *Annals of Allergy, Asthma and Immunology* 105 (2010): 24–30.

Henneberger, P.K., Mirabelli, M.C., Kogevinas, M. *et al.*, 'The occupational contribution to severe exacerbation of asthma', *European Respiratory Journal* 36(2010): 743–750.

Kern, D.G., 'Outbreak of the reactive airways dysfunction syndrome after a spill of glacial acetic acid', *American Review of Respiratory Disease* 144 (1991): 1058–64.

Kronqvist, M., Johansson, E., Kolmodin-Hedman, B. *et al.*, 'IgE-sensitization to predatory mites and respiratory symptoms in Swedish greenhouse workers', *Allergy* 60 (2005): 521–6.

Patiwael, J.A., Jong, N.W., Burdorf, A. *et al.*, 'Occupational allergy to bell pepper pollen in greenhouses in the Netherlands, an eight-year follow-up study', *Allergy* 65 (2010): 1423–9.

Rachiotis, G., Savani, R., Brant, A. *et al.*, 'Outcome of occupational asthma after cessation of exposure: a systematic review', *Thorax* 62 (2007): 147–52.

Schlünssen, V., Kespohl, S., Jacobsen, G. *et al.*, 'Immunoglobulin E-mediated sensitization to pine and beech dust in relation to wood dust exposure levels and respiratory symptoms in the furniture industry', *Scandinavian Journal of Work and Environmental Health* 7 September 2010.

Tagiyeva, N., Devereux, G., Semple, S. *et al.*, 'Parental occupation is a risk factor for childhood wheeze and asthma', *European Respiratory Journal* 35 (2010): 987–93.

Chapter 5

The following is especially useful: G.I. Town, 'Diagnosis in adults', in W.W. Busse and S.T. Holgate (eds) *Asthma and Rhinitis*, Wiley-Blackwell, Oxford second edn, 2008.

Bourke, S.J., *Lecture Notes in Respiratory Medicine*, Blackwell, Oxford, seventh edn 2007.

Coggon, D., Harris, E.C., Brown, T., Rice, S. and Palmer, K.T., 'Work-related mortality in England and Wales, 1979–2000', *Occupational and Environmental Medicine* 67 (2010): 816–22.

Dima, E., Rovina, N., Gerassimou, C. *et al.*, 'Pulmonary function tests, sputum induction, and bronchial provocation tests: diagnostic tools in the challenge of distinguishing asthma and COPD phenotypes in clinical practice', *International Journal of COPD* 5 (2010): 287–96.

Ekici, M., Ekici, A., Keles, H. *et al.*, 'Treatment characteristics in elderly asthmatics', *International Journal of Clinical Practice* 62 (2008): 729–34.

Gibson, P.G., McDonald, V.M. and Marks, G.B., 'Asthma in older adults', *The Lancet* 376 (2010): 803–13.

Hoshino, T., Toda, R. and Aizawa, H., 'Pharmacological treatment in asthma and COPD', *Allergology International* 58 (2009): 341–6.

Lamprecht, B., McBurnie, M.A., Vollmer, W.M. *et al.*, 'COPD in never-smokers: results from the population-based BOLD study', *Chest* (2010) doi: 10.1378/chest.10-1253.

Løkke, A., Lange, P., Scharling, H., Fabricius, P. and Vestbo, J. 'Developing COPD: a 25-year follow-up study of the general population', *Thorax* 61 (2006): 935–9.

McGrath, K.W. and Fahy, J.V., 'Negative methacholine challenge tests in subjects who report physician-diagnosed asthma', *Clinical and Experimental Allergy* 41 (2011): 46–51.

Newman, K.B., Mason, U.G. III and Schmaling, K.B. 'Clinical features of vocal cord dysfunction', *American Journal of Respiratory and Critical Care Medicine* 152 (1995): 1382–6.

NICE (National Institute for Clinical Excellence), *Chronic Obstructive Pulmonary Disease: Management of Chronic Obstructive Pulmonary Disease in Adults in Primary and Secondary Care*, National Clinical Guideline Centre, London 2010; available at <http://guidance.nice.org.uk/CG101/Guidance/pdf/English>.

Núñez, B., Sauleda, J., Antó, J.M. *et al.*, 'Anti-tissue antibodies are related to lung function in chronic obstructive pulmonary disease', *American Journal of Respiratory and Critical Care Medicine* (2010) doi: 10.1164/rccm.201001-0029OC.

Chapter 6

Akpan, A. and Morgan, R., 'Oral candidiasis', *Postgraduate Medical Journal* 78 (2002): 455–9.

Brocklebank, D., Ram, F., Wright, J. *et al.*, 'Comparison of the effectiveness of inhaler devices in asthma and chronic obstructive airways disease: a systematic review of the literature', *Health Technology Assessment* 5 (2001): 26.

Cazzoletti, L., Marcon, A., Janson, C. *et al.*, 'Asthma control in Europe', *Journal of Allergy and Clinical Immunology* 120 (2007): 1360–7.

Clatworthy, J., Price, D., Ryan, D. *et al.*, 'The value of self-report assessment of adherence, rhinitis and smoking in relation to asthma control', *Primary Care Respiratory Journal* 18 (2009): 300–5.

Dore, R.K., 'How to prevent glucocorticoid-induced osteoporosis', *Cleveland Clinic Journal of Medicine* 77 (2010): 529–36.

Gibson, P.G., McDonald, V.M. and Marks, G.B., 'Asthma in older adults', *The Lancet* 376 (2010): 803–13.

Lazarus, S.C., Chinchilli, V.M., Rollings, N.J. *et al.*, 'Smoking affects response to inhaled corticosteroids or leukotriene receptor antagonists in asthma', *American Journal of Respiratory and Critical Care Medicine* 175 (2007): 783–90.

Nyenhuis, S.M., Schwantes, E.A. and Mathur, S.K., 'Characterization of leukotrienes in a pilot study of older asthma subjects', *Immunity and Ageing* 7 (2010): 8.

Suissa, S., Kezouh, A. and Ernst, P., 'Inhaled corticosteroids and the risks of diabetes onset and progression', *American Journal of Medicine* 123 (2010): 1001–6.

Chapter 7

Anon, 'Pandemic influenza: (some) reasons to be cheerful?' *The Lancet* 376 (2010): 565.

Byrne-Davis, L.M.T. and Vedhara, K., 'Psychoneuroimmunology', *Social and Personality Psychology Compass* 2 (2008): 751–64.

Choi, J.Y., Jung, H.J., Kim, J.I. *et al.*, 'A randomized pilot study of acupuncture as an adjunct therapy in adult asthmatic patients', *Journal of Asthma* 47 (2010): 774–80.

Dennis, J., 'Alexander technique for chronic asthma', *Cochrane Database of Systemic Reviews* (2000) CD000995.

Holloway, E.A. and West, R.J., 'Integrated breathing and relaxation training (the Papworth method) for adults with asthma in primary care: a randomised controlled trial', *Thorax* 62 (2007): 1039–42.

Kemeny, M.E., Rosenwasser, L.J., Panettieri, R.A. *et al.*, 'Placebo response in asthma: a robust and objective phenomenon', *Journal of Allergy and Clinical Immunology* 119 (2007): 1375–81.

Loerbroks, A.F., Apfelbacher, C.J., Thayer, J.F. *et al.*, 'Neuroticism, extraversion, stressful life events and asthma: a cohort study of middle-aged adults', *Allergy* 64 (2009): 1444–50.

Mancuso, P. 'Obesity and lung inflammation', *Journal of Applied Physiology* 108 (2010): 722–8.

Ng, T.P., Chiam, P.C. and Kua, E.H., 'Mental disorders and asthma in the elderly: a population-based study', *International Journal of Geriatric Psychiatry* 22 (2007): 668–74.

Schmitz, N., Wang, J. and Malla, A., 'The impact of psychological distress on functional disability in asthma', *Psychosomatics* 50 (2009): 42–9.

Shaw, A., Noble, A., Salisbury, C. *et al.*, 'Predictors of complementary therapy use among asthma patients: results of a primary care survey', *Health and Social Care in the Community* 16 (2008): 155–64.

Sheikh, A., Alves, B. and Dhami, S., 'Pneumococcal vaccine for asthma', *Cochrane Database of Systemic Reviews* (2002) CD002165.

Thomas, M., McKinley, R.K., Mellor, S. *et al.*, 'Breathing exercises for asthma: a randomised controlled trial', *Thorax* 64 (2009): 55–61.

Further reading

Additional information on specific aspects

Baffour, F., *High Risk Body Size: Take control of your weight*. Sheldon Press, London, 2010.

Bradley, D. and Clifton-Smith, T. *Dynamic Breathing: How to manage your asthma*. Sheldon Press, London, 2010.

Delvin, D., *How to Beat Worry and Stress*. Sheldon Press, London, 2010.

Healthcare professionals and biologists may also find the following books useful, which I found invaluable while I was working on this book:

Bourke, S. J., *Lecture Notes in Respiratory Medicine*. Blackwell, Oxford, seventh edn 2007.

Busse, W. W. and Holgate, S. T., *Asthma and Rhinitis*. Blackwell Science, Oxford, second edn 2000.

Kay, A. B., Kaplan, A. P., Bousquet, J. and Holt, P. G. (eds), *Allergy and Allergic Diseases*. Wiley-Blackwell, Oxford, second edn 2008.

I also used the following reviews on several occasions in this book: from *American Family Physician* (*Am Fam Physician*), the *American Journal of Respiratory and Critical Care Medicine* (*Am J Respir Crit Care Med*), the *Canadian Medical Association Journal* (*CMAJ*), the *European Respiratory Journal* (*Eur Respir J*) and the *International Journal of Clinical Practice* (*Int J Clin Pract*):

Balter, M. S., Bell, A. D., Kaplan A. G. *et al.* 'Management of asthma in adults', *CMAJ* 2009; 181:915–22.

Calhoun, W. J., 'Nocturnal asthma', *Chest* (journal of the American College of Chest Physicians) 2003; 123:399S–405S.

Ekici, M., Ekici, A., Keles, H. *et al.* 'Treatment characteristics in elderly asthmatics', *Int J Clin Pract* 2008; 62:729–34.

Gibson, P. G., McDonald, V. M., and Marks, G. B., 'Asthma in older adults', *Lancet* 2010; 376:803–13.

Henneberger, P. K. *et al.*, 'The occupational contribution to severe exacerbation of asthma', *Eur Respir J* 36 2010, 743–50.

Holgate, S. T., Arshad, H. S., Roberts, G. C. *et al.*, 'A new look at the pathogenesis of asthma', *Clinical Science* 2009; 118:439–50.

Kaplan, S. G. *et al.*, 'Diagnosis of asthma in adults', *CMAJ* 2009; 181:E210–20.

Sinha, T. and David, A. K., 'Recognition and management of exercise-induced bronchospasm', *Am Fam Physician* 2003; 67:769–74, 675.

Subbarao, P., Mandhane, P. J., Sears, M. R., 'Asthma: epidemiology, etiology and risk factors', *CMAJ* 2009; 181:E181–90.

Wenzel, S., 'Severe asthma in adults', *Am J Respir Crit Care Med* 2005; 172:149–60.

Index